Childhood Sexual Experiences

Childhood Sexual Experiences

NARRATIVES OF RESILIENCE

SALLY V HUNTER

Senior Lecturer in Health
University of New England
Armidale, New South Wales, Australia

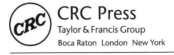

CRC Press
Taylor & Francis Group
Boca Raton London New York

CRC Press is an imprint of the
Taylor & Francis Group, an **informa** business

Radcliffe Publishing Ltd
18 Marcham Road
Abingdon
Oxon OX14 1AA
United Kingdom

www.radcliffe-oxford.com

Electronic catalogue and worldwide online ordering facility.

British Library Cataloguing in Publication Data

A catalogue record for this book is available from the British Library.

ISBN-13: 978 184619 337 8

The paper used for the text pages of this book is FSC certified. FSC (The Forest Stewardship Council) is an international network to promote responsible management of the world's forests.

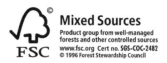

Mixed Sources
Product group from well-managed forests and other controlled sources
www.fsc.org Cert no. SGS-COC-2482
© 1996 Forest Stewardship Council

Typeset by Pindar NZ, Auckland, New Zealand

Contents

About the author

Dr Sally V Hunter was born in the United Kingdom and graduated from Exeter University with a first class honours degree. She migrated to Sydney, Australia in 1986 where she trained as a child and family therapist. She worked in Sydney as a therapist, supervisor and counsellor educator for over 10 years before becoming an academic in rural New South Wales in 2003.

Sally is a Senior Lecturer in Health at the University of New England, Australia. She is an active researcher and author and is well published in her field. She has two adult children of whom she is very proud.

Acknowledgements

This book would not exist without the generosity and openness of the men and women that I interviewed, to whom I am very grateful.

I would also like to acknowledge the support of family, friends and colleagues. In particular I would like to give a warm vote of thanks to my PhD supervisors, Professor Jeffrey Kottler of California State University Fullerton, and Dr Annmaree Wilson of the University of New England, Australia.

I would like to dedicate this book to my three children, Clare, Rosie and James. And to Norman, for changing the narrative of my life so dramatically.

CHAPTER 1

Childhood sexual experiences

INTRODUCTION

Chapter aims
- Introduce the purpose and significance of the research study on which this book is based.
- Locate the author within the topic.
- Challenge readers to review their beliefs about the topic and to see whether or not any of these views are changed by reading this book.

The issue of childhood sexual experiences (CSE) is highly controversial. It is a subject that has generated a complex literature full of disagreement and conflict. The issue is usually framed as child sexual abuse (CSA) and seen as part of the discourse of child maltreatment. Moreover, it is an issue that reflects the social and cultural values of the time and is recognised as a significant social problem.[1]

This book takes an unconventional approach to the topic. It examines the research evidence in a positive manner, and highlights the myriad ways in which people demonstrate their courage and resilience in the face of adversity. It takes a 'glass half full' approach, based on the knowledge that many adults manage to overcome their childhood sexual experiences with adults. It looks at the factors that make people resilient and emphasises these, over and above the risk factors that make people vulnerable. It takes a strength-based approach and explores the narratives that people tell, to themselves and to others about their experiences, which help them to live satisfying lives.

In this book, I have drawn a distinction between *childhood sexual experiences* with adults and *child sexual abuse*. When young children are involved, childhood sexual experiences with adults are always abusive. However, not all people regard their childhood sexual experiences as abusive or are willing to embrace an identity as a victim,[2] and not all believe that their early sexual experiences have had a profoundly negative impact on their lives.[3] This is a book primarily about childhood sexual experiences with adults, *not* a book about child sexual abuse.

Most of the research in the field has been conducted among victims or survivors of child sexual abuse, and this automatically excludes people from the population being studied who are asymptomatic or who demonstrate resilience with regard to childhood sexual experiences.

What makes this book different is that it is *not* based on a clinical sample of survivors of child sexual abuse recruited through clinicians as most other recent qualitative studies have been.

In this study, some of the people interviewed had experienced many years of sexual abuse in childhood, and many years of therapy in adulthood. Others did not necessarily view their childhood sexual experiences as being abusive, or as having a great impact on their lives. Many did not accept what they saw as the stigmatising identity as a victim of child sexual abuse. The study was designed to enable a variety of divergent narratives about childhood sexual experiences, and their meaning and impact, to emerge.[4] It was designed in this way in order to develop a better understanding of resilience and the narratives that people tell about their experiences following childhood maltreatment of this kind.

THE RESEARCH QUESTION

The primary research question that guided this project was: 'what narratives do people tell themselves and others following childhood sexual experiences with adults?' Much of the relevant literature examines the impact of child sexual abuse in terms of adult psychopathology and attempts to determine the factors that influenced the severity of this impact. Little research has been conducted to explain the somewhat challenging findings that some children and adolescents are more severely affected than others by childhood maltreatment,[5] and that some have been able to demonstrate resilience or to be asymptomatic in the face of childhood adversity.[6]

LOCATING THE AUTHOR

Child sexual abuse is often seen as a traumatic experience for a child. I was not sexually abused as a child or as an adult and in that sense I can be seen as an 'outsider' in this research project, with no experience of being victimised. However, this subject matter does touch me deeply on an emotional level because I experienced two traumatic events in my early adulthood. My second daughter died unexpectedly from cot death when she was only 11 weeks old. I then migrated from England to Australia within six months of her death, leaving behind my family and support network. These experiences led me to search for faults in my own behaviour to try to make sense of what had happened.[7] I gradually recovered, and gave birth to my third child. This led me to be strongly connected, and perhaps overprotective, towards my two surviving children. My daughter's death meant that I became a mother first and foremost, and that my career ambitions were placed on hold.

Following my daughter's death, I trained as a feminist systemic therapist and worked as a child and family counsellor in a non-government agency. In this position, I worked with many clients who had experienced child sexual abuse. I became interested in the ways in which they made sense of their experiences. Why were some deeply traumatised by their experiences and yet others appeared to be minimally affected, or even believed that they had grown as a result of the challenges they had faced? I found the capacity of some people to overcome adversity awe-inspiring. In addition, I have always found it hard to comprehend man's inhumanity towards man – or (wo)man's inhumanity towards man, woman and child.

I worked mainly with women, some of whom were in the process of recovering memories of child sexual abuse. A few came into therapy with an already strong sense of self, but most held negative views about themselves as human beings. Challenging these views was often an important part of the therapeutic process. I occasionally felt concerned that my clients were using their therapy sessions in a subtle way to hurt, punish or re-traumatise themselves. I certainly found it challenging to sit with their pain and self-loathing, and with their intense anger and rage at the injustices done to them. The betrayal that many of them faced at the hands of their families was heart-breaking. Working with women who were sexually abused as children touched me personally on two levels: I wanted to reach out and protect the small child within them that had been hurt; and I wanted to reassure myself that adults can survive, overcome traumatic memories and work through feelings of loss and grief.

When working as a therapist, I also saw a lot of couples who were experiencing problems in their sex lives. Now I wonder how many of the men that I met in couples therapy had actually been sexually abused as children but were unwilling or unable to disclose this to their partners. I was not alert to the prevalence of sexual abuse among men and failed to ask deeper questions at the time. The male clients with whom I did discuss sexual abuse tended to move away from the topic fairly quickly and I failed to pursue the issue.

During the length of this research project, many things have happened in my own life. I separated from my long-term partner, decided to put my career first and moved to a rural area living away from my children for the first time. The timing of all these changes was significant – they occurred when my second daughter would have turned 18 had she still been alive. The result has been a painful process of both physical and emotional separation from my two surviving children. Although it was my choice to move away from my family, this separation proved very difficult for me to bear. I underestimated the importance of my day-to-day role as a mother to my sense of self.

These external or public events influenced my internal or private world and vice versa. I moved from a sense of myself as a mother, partner and therapist, to an emerging sense of myself as an academic woman with all that that entails – a role as a teacher, supervisor, colleague and researcher. I gradually adopted a new self-narrative through doing and being – teaching students, discussing issues with colleagues, interviewing participants and listening to and participating in the wider social and cultural debate. My sense of myself as an academic and qualitative researcher has been socially constructed through reflection and interaction with others during this period.

This book was also socially constructed during this time. I moved from a grounded theory approach to a poststructural, narrative approach. I came to see this approach as both an acceptable and a productive way to view such an emotive issue. Taking a social constructionist perspective challenged me not to hide behind a 'truth-based' notion of reality. Instead it encouraged me to reflect on the moral and value-based issues involved and to accept that there is a multiversity of views in relation to complex human, relational experiences.[8]

In writing this book, I became aware that some of the narratives that my participants had told me did not sit comfortably with some of my colleagues. In particular the idea that some participants had not been affected by their early sexual experiences was consistently challenged by others. 'They must be in denial,' or 'Yes, but their stories show how it *has* affected them' was sometimes the response. This was similar to the reactions received by others[9] investigating this topic.

Therapists are encouraged to enter the world of their client, while being aware of their own value systems. However, when dealing with the issue of sexual contact between children and adults, issues of social justice become important and therapists are required to report child maltreatment. It is necessary to take a moral stance over this and other criminal acts involving the use of violence.[10] Taking this stance is justified by the profound impact that childhood sexual experiences can have on children and adolescents. It has never been my intention to argue that childhood sexual experiences are not abusive or that they do not have a profound impact on the lives of some people, or to argue against the moral stance taken by therapists and other health professionals. I share these views and believe that child sexual abuse is a serious crime that needs to be thoughtfully and uncompromisingly dealt with in our society.

However, it has been my intention to open up the possibility of a new dialogue around the issue of childhood sexual experiences, by bringing infrequently heard narratives out into the open. I am using a positive psychology approach to this topic, in the belief that it is useful to hear narratives from people who have demonstrated resilience in the face of adversity or have been able to overcome the difficulties that they have faced.[11] I recognise that taking this approach will pose a challenge to some health professionals reading this book.

THE CHALLENGE TO HEALTH PROFESSIONALS

This book may challenge some of your beliefs, particularly if you have worked extensively with survivors of child sexual abuse who have recovered memories in adulthood. You may have strongly held views about this issue, based on many years of clinical experience working with people who have been severely affected and damaged by their experiences. Many of them will have recovered memories in adulthood and have needed to repress their painful childhood memories through the use of dissociation. It is well known that people who have recovered memories of childhood abuse as adults often suffer tremendously, and may even suffer more distress than those who have continuous memories of abusive experiences from childhood.[12] 'Individuals who report having remembered long-forgotten episodes of CSA are often more psychologically traumatised after recalling the episodes as adults and finally realising that what had happened to them was sexual abuse, than they were when the molestation was occurring during childhood.'[13]

I also held strong views when I started to conduct research in this area but interviewing people has challenged some of these views. And in writing about my research, I hope to challenge your views to a certain extent. However, it is important to remember that many of the participants in this study are different from people that you have met in your consulting room. In this book you will meet people who have talked very little about their childhood sexual experiences and have not sought any treatment. You will meet Greta who saw her childhood sexual experiences as a normal part of her sexual development and under her control. You will meet Peter and Angelo who believed that they were not damaged by their childhood sexual experiences and were able to move on with their lives very successfully. And you will meet Diana, Belinda, Norm, Rod and Will who recognised that they had been severely affected but refused to be viewed as victims, or even as survivors.[14] These people challenged me to consider the issue afresh and to look at the possibility of resilience in the face of adversity, at positive coping through avoidance or denial, and at the difficulty of disclosure and non-disclosure.

Some of these participants were asymptomatic as children and well into adulthood. Some did not find their experiences traumatic at the time or even with hindsight. Some, like Bert, knew that it was socially unacceptable to describe how he had not been negatively affected by his experiences and was reluctant to talk publicly about them for this reason. Of course we cannot assume that an asymptomatic child has not been damaged by child sexual abuse.[15] However, as long ago as the 1980s Finkelhor and his colleagues were asking questions like: 'Is treatment indicated even for children who are showing no symptomatic behaviour?' and 'Can denial be a healthy coping strategy for some children?'[16] They also challenged researchers to determine how the attitudes and feelings differ among those people who had few long-lasting symptoms and demonstrate resilience compared with those who suffered greatly. I would encourage you to read this book with an open mind and to look for the strength and determination to be found in these narratives, remembering that those who are resilient may teach us how better to help those who are less fortunate.

Please answer the questionnaire that follows and keep a record of your answers. Of course there are no right or wrong answers, and many people have very strongly held views on this topic. But some views are based on evidence, whereas others are continually propagated by the media and do not necessarily reflect the 'truth'. Indeed I would argue that there is no one truth, simply many different narratives.

QUESTIONNAIRE

Please answer these questions on a scale from disagree strongly to agree strongly:

Statements about child sexual abuse	Disagree Strongly	Disagree	Neither	Agree	Agree Strongly
	-2	-1	0	+1	+2
1 *All* sexual relationships between children under 16 and adults are forms of child sexual abuse.					
2 Child sexual abuse always has a devastating effect and leads to major mental health problems such as depression and suicidality, self-harm, or sexual problems.					
3 Women find it a lot easier to talk about being sexually abused in childhood than men.					
4 The level of child sexual abuse in a society is linked to the level of poverty.					
5 Most people feel the need to confront their abusers in adulthood, as part of the healing process.					
6 Children often make false accusations about sexual abuse.					
7 When adults recover memories of being sexually abused as children, these memories are always real.					
8 Most people need to relive traumatic childhood experiences before they can move on from them.					
9 I have a sneaking sympathy with those prisoners who 'take the law into their own hands' with convicted paedophiles.					
10 Homosexual men are more likely than heterosexual men to sexually abuse children.					

(continued)

Statements about child sexual abuse	Disagree Strongly	Disagree	Neither	Agree	Agree Strongly
	−2	−1	0	+1	+2
11 The sexual abuse of boys is rare and much less frequent than the sexual abuse of girls.					
12 Boys are usually sexually abused by paedophiles or unknown men, whereas girls are usually abused by their fathers, brothers, stepfathers or men they know.					
13 The present social climate over child sexual abuse is like a witch–hunt in which large numbers of innocent people are bound to be wrongly accused, persecuted and punished.					
14 Sexual abuse of boys by their mothers or sisters is extremely rare.					
15 The emotional damage caused by child sexual abuse is often far worse than any physical hurt or injury.					
16 Sexually abusing children is a psychiatric disorder which requires medical or psychological treatment, rather than imprisonment.					
17 If you have been sexually abused as a child, you are more likely to sexually abuse other children as an adult.					
18 Children often suffer more from being taken away from their families than from the sexual abuse itself.					
19 A consumer society that encourages little girls to buy make-up and adult clothes stimulates the sexual abuse of girl children.					
20 All men who sexually abuse children were sexually abused when they were young.					
21 Men and women who sexually abuse children are callous and feel no remorse.					

Statements about child sexual abuse	Disagree Strongly	Disagree	Neither	Agree	Agree Strongly
	-2	-1	0	+1	+2
22 Fundamentally all forms of child sexual abuse come down to the misuse of adult power over children.					
23 We must not forget that a great deal of suffering that children experience is at the hands of *other children*.					
24 It is naive of therapists to expect sex offenders to take responsibility for their crimes, because they never do.					
25 In child sexual abuse, as for so many other social problems, alcohol abuse has a lot to answer for.					
26 The term 'child abuse' should not be used as a euphemism for acts like rape, buggery and assault.					
27 However worthy the intentions of people like Oprah Winfrey, it is wrong to turn child sexual abuse into entertainment.					
28 Mothers often collude with the sexual abuse of their children, or conveniently 'turn a blind eye'.					
29 What may be sexually abusive in one culture may be considered normal and acceptable behaviour in another.					
30 People can successfully put all thoughts of their childhood sexual abuse out of their minds and lead fulfilling lives, despite their experiences.					

Note: This questionnaire is adapted from statements developed for research.[17]

SUMMARY

Key points

- This is a book primarily about childhood sexual experiences with adults, not about child sexual abuse.
- It takes an unconventional approach by focusing on resilience rather than risk factors.
- It is based on research designed to draw out a variety of narratives about childhood sexual experiences, their meaning and impact.
- It may challenge some of the conventional views held by health professionals about this topic.
- Readers are invited to review their current beliefs about child sexual abuse and to monitor how these are modified, if at all, by reading this book.

In this chapter I have introduced the main purposes and significance of the research project and I have located myself within the topic. I have also challenged readers to review their own beliefs about the topic. The relevant literature will be reviewed and discussed in relation to this project in Chapter 2. The narratives that participants told about their childhood sexual experiences are related in Chapter 3 to Chapter 8. Chapter 9 looks at the issue of disclosure and non-disclosure. This is followed by a discussion in Chapters 10 and 11 and lessons for the future in Chapter 12. Details of the research methodology can be found in the Appendices.

CHAPTER 2

Damaged goods? What we already know about childhood sexual experiences

INTRODUCTION

Chapter aims
- Describe what the current literature tells us about child sexual abuse and childhood sexual experiences.
- Estimate how many people have childhood sexual experiences with adults and their potential impact on the person.
- Identify the extent to which the family and environmental factors can be protective and risk factors.

In this chapter I briefly describe what the current literature tells us about the issue of child sexual abuse and childhood sexual experiences. I examine the prevalence of child sexual abuse and its long-term effects, and the protective and risk factors including the family environment and other influences such as cultural differences. A more detailed literature review has been reported elsewhere.[1]

The focus of this chapter is on the experiences of adults who were sexually abused in childhood, rather than on the experiences of families in which a child has recently disclosed sexual abuse, or on victimisers. I have deliberately taken a positive approach to the statistics, in order to offer a more balanced approach to the topic than those based on what has been called *survivor-based knowledge*. In doing so, I do not wish to undermine the genuine suffering experienced by many people who have had childhood sexual experiences. Neither do I want to minimise the potential impact of such offensive behaviour. My aim is to offer an alternative view to those commonly found in the current literature.

Below is one example of the negative approach used in the literature in this field. In Sanderson's book on counselling adult survivors of child sexual abuse, she lists the potential negative consequences for the adult survivor. Although these symptoms are all possible outcomes of child sexual abuse, the list quickly becomes overwhelming to the reader and does little to engender hope for a full recovery in adulthood:

> Damaged self-structures also lead to feelings of hopelessness, powerlessness, sense of betrayal and defilement, disposition to self-abuse, detachment and loss of bonding capacity, external locus of control and impaired socialization. These in turn give rise to demoralization, dispiritedness, existential doubt of meaning of life, loss of stability and continuity, fragmentation of identity, identity disturbance and diffusion, shame, self-doubt, loss, self-destructive tendencies, and suicidal tendencies.[2]

There is another way to look at the statistics since not all children experience all of these negative outcomes. In fact, many children and adults show no symptoms at all. This chapter presents a more balanced picture of the range of possible outcomes following childhood sexual experiences with adults.

THE PREVALENCE OF CHILD SEXUAL ABUSE AND CHILDHOOD SEXUAL EXPERIENCES

It is very difficult to give an accurate picture of the frequency with which child sexual abuse occurs. There are no common definitions in the literature and, with such an emotive topic, it is difficult to estimate the accuracy of the statistics that are collected. We know that most people choose not to disclose that they have been sexually abused as children until well into adulthood and that men are less likely to make disclosures than women. Hence reliable statistics in this field are difficult to find. What we do know is that child sexual abuse is far more common than we would like to believe and that it frequently occurs within families and stepfamilies or with someone that is known to the child, rather than being perpetrated by an unknown person or a paedophile.

Much sexual abuse remains hidden from view. In a UK study conducted among young people, about 10% reported experiencing behaviour as children that the interviewer rated as sexual abuse involving physical contact of some kind.[3] As is commonly reported, the percentage was higher for girls (15%) than for boys (6%). The overall figure may be an underestimate because a further 6% described consensual sexual behaviour when aged between 13 and 15 with someone five or more years older. Adding these figures together gives a total of 16% of young people being assessed as having experienced sexual abuse involving physical contact as children. However, only 6% of them described their experiences as being sexually abused – an example of the under-reporting that occurs.

In Australia the data is similar with 10% of women and 3% of men claiming to have been forced or frightened into unwanted sexual activity under the age of 16.[4] Overall 13% of women and 21% of men claimed to have had consensual sex before that age too. Most researchers agree that more young girls than boys are sexually abused, whereas more young boys than girls claim to have consensual sex before the age of consent. We also know that men are less likely than women to disclose having been sexually abused, for fear of the stigmatisation attached to homosexual experiences and the shame attached to heterosexual experiences. So it is possible that the figures for men are far closer to those for women than is currently believed. It is also emerging that the sexual abuse of young boys by women is far more common than previously believed and may even be more common than the sexual abuse of boys by men, although these occurrences are much more likely to be described by the young boy as consensual.[5]

THE LONG-TERM IMPACT OF CHILD SEXUAL ABUSE

There is evidence that, for some people, the experience of child sexual abuse has a profound impact on their lives. This impact on mental health and well-being has been extensively described. There is a correlation between being sexually abused as a child and experiencing serious problems in adult life. However, there is not a one-to-one correspondence between child maltreatment and problems in adulthood, and many people who have childhood sexual experiences with adults remain asymptomatic into adulthood. It remains difficult to predict who will suffer most, although there is some evidence that distress varies with a number of factors, such as the severity of the abuse and the victim's relationship with the victimiser, with the closer the relationship, the more distress experienced. It is also difficult to predict which children will remain asymptomatic and be less affected than others by their childhood sexual experiences.

The topic of child sexual abuse evokes strong emotional responses in people which are reflected in media coverage of the topic. This makes it very difficult to give a balanced picture, because any suggestion other than that it does irreparable harm to the child involved is likely to be condemned as supporting paedophilia.[6] However, to say that childhood sexual experiences do not always cause intense harm to the child is different from saying that sexual contact between adults and children is acceptable behaviour. Clearly, it is not.

The particular types of problems in adulthood that have been related to child sexual abuse are depression, alcohol abuse, antisocial behaviour, suicide risk, anxiety about sex, personal problems such as increased numbers of divorces, increased likelihood of unfaithfulness within relationships, and increased risk of re-victimisation among men and women. There is also evidence of problems with intimacy and sexual functioning among men. A correlation between child sexual abuse and the development of substance abuse problems in adolescence has also been shown, although the link between these in not well understood. The impact of child sexual abuse and the subsequent choices made by the young person often reverberate well into adulthood, with far-reaching consequences.

It is certainly true that adults who were sexually abused as children are about four times more likely to have contact with mental health service providers than the general population.[7] A relatively small percentage (12%) of people who have been sexually abused as children go on to develop severe mental health problems later in life (admittedly three times higher than the level found in the general population). Only a small percentage of their problems can be directly attributed to their child sexual abuse rather than to other factors in their lives. Thus, although the likelihood of developing a severe mental health problem is higher for an adult who was sexually abused as a child, most (88%) do not develop severe problems or seek treatment. Other factors, such as the family, cultural or socioeconomic environment can also act as either protective or risk factors for the child.

There is a large number of variables that may influence the impact that child sexual abuse has on the individual child. These variables are interwoven and include the age and sex of the child, the nature of the relationship between the adult and the child, the severity of the abuse, use of force or coercion, other forms of maltreatment experienced by the child, and the frequency and duration of the abuse. Whether or not the experience was heterosexual or homosexual in nature may influence the likelihood of disclosure and help-seeking. This makes it very difficult to predict the effects, outcomes and long-term consequences of childhood sexual experiences for an individual child.

As many as 40% of children who have been sexually abused have few or no symptoms on standard measurements.[8] This became known as the issue of 'the asymptomatic child'. Many clinicians were puzzled by this phenomenon and were unable to decide whether or not these children were in denial. It has been suggested that there could be a sleeper effect, and these children might go on to develop mental health problems in adulthood.

In the 1980s feminist researchers argued that it was important to view child sexual abuse on a continuum along with pornography, rape and other forms of male violence such as domestic violence.[9] Others have argued that it is more useful to place child sexual abuse on a continuum with family violence and family dysfunction in general.[10] Certainly, the family environment can often be seen as either protective or a further risk factor for the child.

PROTECTIVE AND RISK FACTORS IN THE FAMILY ENVIRONMENT

Child maltreatment often goes hand in hand with other life challenges, such as poverty or living in an unsupportive family environment. This makes it difficult to isolate the impact of child sexual abuse from these other factors. However, this also offers encouragement to families and to clinicians working with families where an incident of child sexual abuse occurs in the context of an otherwise well functioning family. A good family environment may not be able to prevent child sexual abuse, but it will help to protect the child from the negative consequences of their experiences.

Unfortunately, children who experience child sexual abuse often grow up in non-protective family environments. Many experience other forms of child maltreatment as well, such as emotional abuse, neglect, physical abuse, or the witnessing of domestic violence in the home.[11] Abuse by siblings and peers is believed to be more common than is currently realised, particularly in dysfunctional families.[12] The family environment,[13] the level of parental functioning[14] and experiencing other forms of child maltreatment[15] have all been shown to be risk factors in child sexual abuse and correlated with negative outcomes in adult life. Sadly, family dysfunction and other forms of child maltreatment often form the context within which child sexual abuse occurs, and physical abuse is frequently used or threatened as a coercive tactic to enforce the child's silence.[16]

It is important to remember that a statistical correlation does not prove a causal relationship. We need to consider whether family dysfunction leads to child sexual abuse or vice versa. For example, children have been shown to be more vulnerable to child sexual abuse following parental separation when they are living with single parents. However, it is also possible that child sexual abuse may have been the cause of the parental separation; hence the statistical correlation found.[17] Parental attitudes to what has happened may also be very important influences on the long-term recovery of the child.

Notifications of child maltreatment happen across the social spectrum, although they are disproportionately high for economically disadvantaged populations in the United States,[18] the United Kingdom[19] and Australia.[20] Those living in poverty and, in particular Indigenous Australians, have higher levels of ill health including mental health problems such as addictions, higher levels of unemployment, higher levels of incarceration and poorer housing, lower average incomes and lower levels of participation and achievement in education[21] to name but a few knock-on effects of poverty. Indigenous Australians also experience higher levels of child sexual abuse, particularly those living within remote Aboriginal communities.[22]

DIFFERENCES BY CULTURE OR ETHNIC GROUP

There are also known differences in terms of what would be considered child maltreatment across cultures as suggested by the worldwide variability in the age of consent.[23] The literature suggests that children are sexually abused at relatively comparable rates across cultures, with minor variations. No consistent cultural variations have been found in relation to the severity of child sexual abuse, the disclosure of such abuse, or in terms of emotional responses to child maltreatment. Most studies have examined differences across broad ethnic groups only, such as African-Americans, and have not explored issues such as acculturation or the extent to which strong protective cultural values have been transmitted down the generations.

In the US children of African-American, Native American, or Latino descent are significantly over-represented in the child protection and foster care systems[24] This is either as a result of institutional discrimination or other risk factors such as low socioeconomic status, living in relatively dangerous neighbourhoods, living in single-parent families or in families with more than four children, or with unemployed caregivers.[25]

There is a similar pattern found in Australia where Aboriginal and Torres Strait Islander children are six times more likely than non-Indigenous children to have an allegation of child maltreatment substantiated in their family.[26] Having said that, there is probably a high level of denial about the extent of child maltreatment within Aboriginal communities.[27] The issue is complicated by racism, historical oppression and lack of trust in government departments by Aboriginal people following the systematic removal of Aboriginal children from their families throughout the last century, known as the Stolen Generations.[28]

Some cultural backgrounds bring with them both greater risks and greater protective factors.[29] For example, African-American communities often have stronger bonds and social fabric that may help to protect children from sexual abuse. However, African-American children may suffer more serious consequences as a result of child sexual abuse because of systemic discrimination, living in poverty, potential stigmatisation and lack of culturally appropriate services.[30] In Australia many Aboriginal and Torres Strait Islander children, particularly those in remote communities, live in poverty as a result of structural inequality. Given the strong relationship between poverty and child abuse and neglect, this places them at risk despite many protective Indigenous cultural values. This may be one of the main reasons for the over-representation of Indigenous children in the child protection system.[31]

SUMMARY

Key points
- Child sexual abuse occurs across all socioeconomic and cultural groups.
- Much remains hidden from view, partly because not all people identify their childhood sexual experiences as abusive and partly because there are many barriers to disclosure.
- It is possible that the prevalence of sexual abuse of boys is almost as high as that of girls, but boys are less likely to disclose sexual abuse than girls.
- Children of colour and Indigenous children are over-represented in official statistics despite protective cultural values, possibly because of the strong correlation between poverty and child maltreatment.
- Child sexual abuse can have a devastating impact and is correlated with poor mental health outcomes in adulthood.
- The severity of the impact varies according to numerous interwoven factors.
- As many as 40% of children remain asymptomatic following child sexual abuse and 88% do not seek treatment in adulthood.
- The main risk factors that increase the negative impact of child sexual abuse include poverty and deprivation, family dysfunction, poor parenting and experiencing other forms of child maltreatment. It is hard to determine whether family dysfunction leads to child sexual abuse or vice versa.
- Coming from a minority group or different ethnic background may be either a protective or a risk factor in relation to child sexual abuse.

In this chapter I have summarised the research evidence in relation to the prevalence of child sexual abuse and childhood sexual experiences. I have examined the factors that influence the likely impact of these experiences on the child and discussed the possibility of children remaining asymptomatic. I have also looked at the risk and the protective factors including the family environment and possible cultural influences.

The prevalence of child sexual abuse is far greater than it should be across all societies and cultures. It often coexists with structural poverty and deprivation. It has a variable impact that is difficult to predict. Researchers continue to search for both risk and protective factors that influence the resilience of people who have had these experiences.

Government health warning!

I feel the need to warn you that some of the stories that follow make grim reading and may be distressing to some readers. I have included some of the graphic descriptions of what happened to these people when they were children. I have not included this material to titillate the reader or to sensationalise the topic. Rather I have included it because I think it is important to know what type of childhood sexual experiences we are talking about and how these men and women have managed to overcome them.

These stories have been presented as they were told to me in the interview and as if they were real events that actually happened. Given the reconstructive nature of memories, it is not possible to determine whether or not they were in fact real events, or reconstructed in adulthood from real or imagined memories of childhood events. Most people seemed convinced most of the time that they were describing events that had actually happened to them in reality. Whenever they expressed uncertainty about the veracity of their memories this has been noted.

The first narrative is the *narrative of normal sexual development.* Given that I interviewed people for about two hours on average, the material presented here represents a small fraction of what they said during that time. Inevitably, I have had to condense their stories, and have chosen to focus on particular aspects of interest in relation to the development of a resilient narrative about childhood sexual experiences. I have used their exact words, edited and reordered to make a more flowing narrative. However, I have given each person a pseudonym and protected their identity by changing non-essential details of their stories.

CHAPTER 3

Normal sexual development

INTRODUCTION

> **Chapter aims**
> - Tell the narrative of two men and women who saw their childhood sexual experiences as part of the normal sexual development process.
> - Describe their belief that they were unharmed by these experiences.
> - Explain the factors that may have helped them to be resilient.

This chapter focuses on the stories told by two people, Greta and Bert, who saw their childhood sexual experiences as part of the normal process of sexual development, even though they would be defined by legal systems all over the world as sexually abusive. This is a somewhat controversial narrative, given that their experiences were clearly sexually abusive. However, both were motivated to tell their stories because they honestly believed that they hadn't been badly affected by their childhood sexual experiences and that other people who have similar experiences would be relieved to hear their stories. They wanted others to know that it was possible to have a sexual experience in childhood without being so damaged by it that it affected the outcome of your whole life. They were both what has been described in the literature as asymptomatic children,[1] which begs the question as to whether or not they were unharmed or the effects of such harm were subtle and delayed. They certainly believed the former, i.e. that they were unharmed by the child maltreatment that they experienced.

NOT BEING AFFECTED

Both Greta and Bert thought of their childhood sexual experiences as an exciting part of their normal sexual development in adolescence. Each felt that these experiences had neither a positive nor a negative effect on their lives. They didn't believe that they had experienced any serious problems as a result of these events in childhood and had never felt the need for therapy in relation to them. Deciding whether or not to tell anyone about what happened was a non-issue because they felt no need to do so.

Greta's story – 'unloading my virginity'

Greta was a woman in her mid-forties, married with two children, and working as a professional in a small country town. Greta was highly intelligent but was given no encouragement to achieve at school or to better herself, since her parents didn't have very high expectations for her. They lived in a small rural community, where she had exploratory sexual experiences with the boy next door and with a girl of about her age when she was 13. She felt there was nothing for her at home so she moved out as soon as she could, at the age of 15, to get a job and to explore the world.

Shortly after leaving home, Greta had sexual intercourse with a 25-year-old man. She liked him, but she wasn't emotionally involved with him. She felt in control of the situation and there had been no negative consequences – she didn't get pregnant or feel pressured to have sex with him again. She had satisfied her curiosity about what it was like to have sexual intercourse.

She talked about this experience to her girlfriends but not to her parents, whom she didn't see for a year after she left home. It was as if it was part of an individuation process for her. Choosing to have sex was an important symbol of her new-found independence from her family and of standing on her own two feet. She saw it as an appropriate way to begin her sex life and was proud of how she had behaved.

This is Greta's story, told in her own words.

> I saw myself as a virgin until I was 15. And by that time I had left home. We lived way out in the country, and it was a very isolated, backwater community, a bit of a hillbilly community. And I was really desperate to leave because there was nothing there and it was terribly restrictive. But I was very interested in sex and was quite keen to try it out.
>
> I lost my virginity with a man who would have been 10 years older than me. I had sex with him in the back seat of his car when I was drunk, but I never felt that he had taken advantage of me. It was like something that I was keen to do. And he seemed like the person to do it with. Firstly, because I liked him and felt sexually attracted to him. But also because I wasn't having a relationship with him, there wasn't an emotional connection there, except that I thought he was a nice bloke. But I wasn't in love with him, if that makes sense. And that suited me, because I didn't want that complication. But I wanted to try sex out, and I trusted him. But I was a bit shy, so being a bit drunk was a good thing for me as well. So it was kind of almost engineered. And I only had sex with that guy

once but that suited me well too. I wanted to unload my virginity. I had been thinking about sex, you know, for a number of years and I was keen to do it and that's really all there was to it.

As Greta was talking, I was thinking about how different her experience was from those of the other men and women I had interviewed. She believed that she had been in control of the situation and had made a choice to have sexual intercourse. As the interview went on, she realised that she had trusted this particular man, even though he hadn't used a condom and she wasn't on the pill.

And the impact, I didn't think much of it at the time, still don't really. It's just what happened to me. I didn't ever feel that I was coerced into sex, or that people took advantage of me. I felt I was responsible for what I did. And I felt to some degree in control of what that was, what I was after, and I never felt that people had persuaded me to do something that I didn't want to do, or that I was abused, or anything really. In fact I feel a bit proud that that's the way I did things and I think it's an appropriate way to begin my sexual life. So that was what I wanted at the time, that was my choice, it worked out the way I expected, there were no repercussions or problems.

There was no sense that Greta saw herself as the victim of an older predatory male. In fact she went on to describe some of the positive things that she gained from her early sexual experiences with both men and women.

So I guess the positive things are that I had the opportunity to think about sex in a range of ways. And also having some of my first sexual experiences with another woman, or another girl, we were only very young at the time, also was a more broad way of thinking about sex than just the traditional. So I think that sort of gave me a bit more of a different insight into sex, and I've had sex with women since then. I think that's positive as well. It gives you just a broader way of looking at your sexual life. So all of those early experiences actually were, they weren't with strangers, they were with people that I knew, that I had some sort of relationship with, that I felt safe with, that I trusted. I've never thought about that before, but now I think through it, I think that's an important part, that kind of safety.

Greta felt good about choosing to have sexual intercourse at that time in her life and about the way that it had happened. For her, it was a liberating experience that symbolised her new-found ability to stand on her own two feet and to live independently from her parents.

We were taught that you didn't have sex until you got married, and if you did, then you were a tart. And I think my father would have seen my behaviour as I was a tart. So there was that kind of climate, but he never would have talked to me about sex except to be furious if I had gotten pregnant ever. My mother would have been upset, but I think she was more understanding. So part of all this was leaving home, and getting away from that home environment. There was nothing there. There was no encouragement, there was no anything. I guess it was an interesting part of my life and it was certainly an exciting part of my life.

It seemed to me that Greta chose to have sexual intercourse with a man she liked and trusted and with whom she felt safe. She saw this as a form of sexual experimentation, which she felt no shame or guilt about. She didn't believe that having sex at that age had a great deal of impact on her life, and rarely thought about it. She was proud of the way that she handled herself and, despite the 10-year age gap, she didn't feel that she had been coerced into having sex in any way. Perhaps because there were no perceived negative outcomes for her, she felt comfortable about what had happened.

Protective factors contributed to Greta's resilience

I believe that there were certain individual, family and environmental protective factors that buffered Greta and helped her to be resilient in this situation. By resilience I mean that she was able to 'function well in spite of adverse experiences, of relative resistance to risk factors, or of overcoming stress experiences'.[2] She was a highly intelligent young woman who enjoyed a reasonable level of family support in that her parents were not highly abusive towards her[3] and had reasonable parenting skills.[4] Even at a young age resilient children and adolescents are less reactive to stress, less emotional and less aggressive than non-resilient children and seem to be able to select or construct for themselves supportive environments, by seeking the help and support they need from others.[5] Greta seemed able to do this for herself, by choosing to leave home at 15, move in with friends, find a job and support herself.

I have met other young people who, like Greta, believed that their childhood sexual experiences were perfectly normal and healthy despite being under the age of consent and with a much older person. This is a criminal offence in Australia, and in many other countries, and yet Greta did not experience it as abusive or traumatic. She is one of many young people who have sexual experiences under the age of consent with people at least five years older than themselves but which they consider to be consensual. She took the experience in her stride at the time, didn't dwell on it negatively and moved on with life. Bert was able to do much the same.

Bert's story – 'like pinching apples'

Bert was in his late forties and lived in a small rural town. He worked part-time and looked after his two adolescent children, following a separation from his wife. Bert described growing up in a strict, religious household where talking about sex was strictly taboo and homosexuality simply didn't exist. When he was 11 he had four sexual encounters with a male family friend.

Bert wasn't disturbed by what happened. In fact, he found it quite interesting at the time. He wanted to be interviewed because he thought that these experiences hadn't harmed him. He knew that this was a totally unacceptable thing to say publicly in the current climate. During the interview, he seemed relieved to be able to talk in a more open and honest manner.

Bert started a five-year homosexual relationship with a boy of his own age when he was 14. He then had a long-term heterosexual relationship in his twenties and thirties, and now describes himself as bisexual. He didn't believe that his childhood experiences had any impact on his sexuality. He thought that they might have made him more interested in sex from an early age, partially explaining why he entered a homosexual relationship with a boy of his own age at 14. However, he didn't see this as negative. This is how he told his story.

> Well, it's not a long story. As far as I can remember I was about 10 or 11, and there was a man who would drive me home after an extra-curriculum activity. When he drove me home, he exposed himself, he had an erection, he masturbated, he wanted me to masturbate him, and he wanted me to undress, which I did. And for some short time, 10 minutes, 15 minutes, and then we'd get dressed and he'd drop me home. And then the next week, the same thing happened, maybe three or four times. He was a friend of the family. They went to the same church, good church-going people, seems to be a prerequisite requirement actually. He didn't force me and he didn't threaten me. Nevertheless, I did keep it secret. I didn't tell anyone at the time, and I didn't tell anyone at all until I was married.
>
> I remember not being particularly traumatised or anything of that sort. I remember thinking 'that was kind of interesting'. I knew that it was some sort of transgression, but it was a minor one to my mind. It's like you and your mate are going to jump over a fence and pinch apples off someone's tree, and you know it's naughty. You know you shouldn't do it, but it's not a capital offence, it's a minor thing. And having jumped over the fence and pinched the apples, you share that secret with the other person. So you have a bond with this other person because you've done this transgression together. And if I didn't tell, and he didn't tell, then we had that bond.

I was impressed with the way that Bert spoke about his experiences. He spoke slowly and weighed his words carefully. He wanted to explain clearly how he felt at the time. It was as if he shared a secret with this man. He felt curious about what had happened, rather than disgusted or frightened by it. He certainly didn't feel traumatised by in any way.

> I felt like the selected one, because he's selected me. He was in control; I mean he was an adult. I was 11; he was a grown-up. And when grown-ups tell you to do stuff, well, they're adults, so you have to. There's a simple, complete power thing. So he didn't actually force me, but just the fact that he was an adult and I was a child meant that I complied. And I think I wanted to comply because he was letting me in on this secret. I was sort of manipulated into doing it, but I didn't feel manipulated at the time. It was physically pleasurable and it was interesting, like it was 'Wow'. It was like 'Oh'. It was like a discovery.
>
> Because I'd complied, I hadn't fought tooth and nail, in my mind I was guilty of the transgression. So if I'd told my parents then I would've been in strife, because I was guilty of doing it. Now looking back, if I had've told them, it could've been completely different. I don't know. Although knowing my parents, they probably would've denied that any such thing was ever possible, and they probably would've done nothing, I dare say. Maybe that's why I didn't tell them. It was actually safer to keep it a secret than to be open about it.

For Bert, keeping secrets became a habit. I thought that this might partly be because he identified as bisexual and therefore needed to be secretive about his sexuality. He knew that his parents would not be able to accept that he was homosexual and had never even tried to tell them.

> Sex was an absolutely taboo subject in our house, of any sort. Sex was never, ever discussed at any time in our house. And homosexuality, well, you can forget that because that didn't even exist as far as within our household. You just deny any of that stuff happened. So talking about it to my parents was just impossible really because I would have been punished for bringing the subject up. And in any case, I didn't think that they'd have any understanding of what I was talking about because they'd never talked about it. As far as I knew, they didn't know anything about sex or homosexuality or sexual assault.

Without being asked the question, Bert explained that he didn't believe that his homosexual experience at the age of 11 had affected his sexuality. He conceded, however, that it might have made him sexually precocious at a younger age.

> I did have a homosexual relationship for five years, starting when I was 14, with someone my age. So even at 14 I'd actually decided that I was homosexual, and that was just a statement of fact, that was just it. And then around about 19, 20, well, 18, 19, 20, 21, I started to wonder about whether that was right, and I sort

of went straight after that. I don't think that that episode, or those three or four goes with that man, I don't think that made my sexual orientation change. No. I think it was probably wired well before that, and that just happened. I don't think that caused any sort of change in my sexual orientation. I think it might've made me more – what's the word? – precocious, in the sense that I might not have been sexually active so young if that hadn't happened, maybe.

It is inevitable that some of you will be questioning whether or not Bert was denying the impact of his childhood sexual experiences on him. I wondered about the same issue at the time. But Bert insisted that his experiences were non-traumatic and just one part of life's rich tapestry. He knew that this is an unacceptable point of view these days and one that he was unable to express publicly. He was relieved to be able to tell me openly that he had been sexually abused as a child and that he was okay, without being accused of siding with paedophiles or even of being one himself.

> I don't think it had a great effect actually, I really don't. I certainly don't, I've never sat and mulled about it. It doesn't go round and round in my head. I've never really discussed it openly with friends that I trust, and the reason is that I'm afraid of their reaction. Because I don't think that I've been traumatised by this event. And if I say that, people's reaction will be 'Oh, so you think it was okay to do that. So you think it's okay for adults to coerce children into having sex, because it actually doesn't hurt them.' And I don't think that at all, but people will conclude that. But I'm actually sort of okay. But this is the only time I've ever said this, which I have to tell you is a great relief [laughs] to actually to say it, that it's not okay, but I don't think that I was really hurt by it. It's just something that happened.

Both Greta and Bert saw their childhood sexual experiences as part of their normal sexual development. However, unlike Greta, Bert did feel somewhat guilty about what he had done. He chose to keep both the incidents and his sexuality a secret from his parents. This was an important contradiction that ran through Bert's narrative – he sincerely believed that what had happened had not affected him, and yet he also felt guilty and chose to keep silent about these events.

Bert's pattern of secrecy

I was particularly struck by the way in which societal beliefs had silenced Bert as an adult. He was very reluctant to talk publicly about his sexual experiences for fear that others might judge him to be, at best, weird and, at worst, a potential paedophile. He was genuinely concerned that he would be seen to be advocating sex between adults and children, if he spoke honestly about his belief that he had not been negatively affected by his experiences.

Bert learned to keep secrets from his parents at a young age, as many children do. He used what has been termed avoidant coping or motivated forgetting from his early childhood. This has been described as a maladaptive or risky strategy,[6] which may lead to symptoms of psychological distress and to more severe problems in adulthood. However, it has also been seen as a functional and appropriate coping mechanism and a useful way of avoiding dwelling on unpleasant memories or thoughts.

Bert's story was complicated by the fact that Bert was bisexual, another fact that he chose to keep secret from his parents. Young gay men often don't identify their childhood sexual experiences with older men as sexually abusive or they choose to believe that they were the ones to initiate the experience.[7] It is possible that some young gay men believe that it is safer to make a sexual advance towards an older man than towards another adolescent and risk being rejected, hurt or even outed as a result.[8]

Ever since Freud and Breuer first described the defence mechanism of repression as a way of pushing an inconceivable idea from the conscious mind,[9] there has been a debate about whether or not such an action is a useful and functional coping mechanism or a maladaptive form of denial. In terms of child sexual abuse, the question becomes: 'Can denial be a healthy coping strategy for some children?'[10] Secrecy certainly seemed to work well for Bert. This form of avoidant coping is also apparent in the stories told in the next chapter.

NARRATIVE OF NORMAL SEXUAL DEVELOPMENT

I have termed this a *narrative of normal sexual development*. This is a resilient narrative told by two people who held the somewhat surprising view that they had not been damaged by their childhood sexual experiences with adults. Indeed Greta and Bert believed that their early sexual experiences were not abusive and were an exciting part of their normal sexual development. They felt little guilt about what had happened and the issue of telling or not telling seemed largely irrelevant to them. They both described themselves as curious about sex from a young age and had both had heterosexual and homosexual experiences in adolescence. Both knew that it was not culturally acceptable to talk about not being affected in today's climate of 'moral panic'[11] relating to sex crimes and paedophilia. Greta stood out in that she did not view her childhood sexual experiences as in any way abusive, even as an adult, and believed that she had been in control of what had happened.

In this chapter I have explored the narrative of *normal sexual development*. In the next chapter, I will describe the narrative of *a silence recently broken*. This is a similar narrative in that the men and women telling it also believed that they had not been badly affected by their childhood sexual experiences.

SUMMARY

Key points

- This narrative challenges the idea that all childhood sexual experiences with adults are always considered harmful by the child involved.
- Both Greta and Bert saw what happened to them as part of their normal sexual development and in no way harmful to them.
- Both grew up in relatively well functioning families and were not physically or emotionally abused at home.
- Greta believed that she had been in control of what happened to her, and both she and Bert were slightly older when the sexual experiences occurred.
- It is important to consider whether or not Greta and Bert were in denial, were using avoidant coping mechanisms to good effect, or were not traumatised by their experiences as they themselves believed to be the case.
- It is interesting to note that both Greta and Bert described themselves as sexually curious from a young age.

CHAPTER 4

A silence recently broken

INTRODUCTION

Chapter aims
- Tell the narratives of four men and women who have recently broken their silence about their childhood sexual experiences.
- Describe their controversial and socially unacceptable belief that they were not badly affected by these experiences.
- Explain their contradictory feelings of shame and self-blame.
- Illustrate how they coped by deciding not to think about these events.
- Outline how they are beginning to see their experiences in a new light as having had an impact on their intimate relationships.
- Describe some of their concerns about the impact that their childhood experiences may have had on their sexual behaviour as adults.

This chapter focuses on the lives of four people who told of *a silence recently broken*. This title has been deliberately chosen to reflect the contradictory nature of their narratives. Even though these men and women believed that they chose to keep silent about their childhood sexual experiences, they volunteered to be interviewed and had eventually disclosed what had happened to them. Jim summed up the essence of these narratives when he said: 'Silence was how I talked about it.'

The four people telling or, for a long time, not telling *narratives of a silence recently broken* believed that their childhood sexual experiences hadn't had a negative impact on their lives and, hence, there was no need for them to talk about it. Victoria, Angelo, Jim and Peter recognised that their childhood sexual experiences were out of the ordinary, but they believed that they had been able to move on with their lives without any apparent ill effect and without needing to talk about it to anyone else.

Why would someone volunteer for a study if they have never spoken about their childhood sexual experiences before? Why would they volunteer if they believed that these experiences hadn't affected them? This chapter unpacks the complicated reasons why these people came forward to tell their stories at that particular point in their lives.

NO NEGATIVE IMPACT EXCEPT ON INTIMATE LIVES

Victoria, Angelo, Jim and Peter recognised that what had happened to them as children had been unusual. Despite feeling some shame, they all reported moving on successfully with their lives and seemed to have deliberately chosen not to think about what had happened to them. Recently, as discussion of paedophilia and child sexual abuse had become more common in the Australian media, they had started to reconsider their experiences and to wonder whether or not they had been affected more than they originally thought, particularly in relation to their sex lives. Perhaps as a result, they had decided to break the silence and come forward to be interviewed.

Victoria's story – 'in good hands'

Victoria invited her sister, Tess, to attend the interview with her. Both young women had slightly different stories to tell and were sometimes surprised by what the other had said. Victoria described how her childhood had been very happy until her stepfather had arrived on the scene. Her parents had an open marriage and initially they lived in a *ménage à trois*. Victoria just accepted the idea that she was lucky to have two fathers. She was introduced to sexual behaviour at a very young age, in a highly sexualised family environment. Her mother and stepfather frequently had sex in front of her. The two adults planned that he would have penetrative sex with Victoria for the first time on her sixteenth birthday.

Victoria was very frightened when this happened and she cried. Following this incident, her stepfather started to have penetrative sex with her 14-year-old sister Tess. Victoria claimed that things were tougher for Tess, although she seemed uncertain as to what had actually happened to her, as if she was experiencing some amnesia. Of the two sisters, she seemed to be much more able to put it out of her mind.

Victoria was frightened of her mother, and she had lived at home until she got married at age 26. She believed that her mother loved her stepfather unreservedly and had, therefore, been willing to go along with what he wanted. She didn't see her mother's behaviour as abusive, just as loving towards him. She was frightened that she might make the same mistake herself, by falling in love with a sexually abusive man who would hurt her daughter.

We had a fantastic, a fantastic childhood. Mum was fun, she was fantastic. I was like her best friend. My mum and dad had an open marriage. Our mother is a liar [laughs]. There was always boyfriends. Even when the stepfather came on the scene, Dad, the stepfather and Mum, we all lived together. Like Mum and Dad had a room upstairs, and Jon and Mum had a room downstairs. So it was a very weird set-up, but it didn't feel weird at the time. It was kind of like 'cool'. It was like 'We have two dads and they live with us.' She was madly, madly in love with Jon. He was the love of her life.

I felt shocked and saddened as Victoria and her sister described the extraordinary behaviour of their mother, father and stepfather. Victoria seemed to have very little understanding of what had really been going on. It was hard for me, as a mother myself, to understand how Victoria's mother could have condoned the sexual abuse of her own daughters and could decide to have sexual intercourse in front of them.

I can remember laying there, as stiff as a board, and they were discussing in bed, with me there. Mum was saying, 'Yes, I'd like it if you were the first, because that way I'd know she'd be in good hands.' At one stage they were discussing me having his baby, because she couldn't have any more children [sighs]. When he and I were having intercourse, she wasn't there. She was either at the pub or at work. But while they were having sex, I was normally in the bed. But I didn't get it as bad as Tess, because he tried to penetrate me and it hurt too much. And he must've got put off because I was crying and that, and then he didn't really try after that, it was more just touching, feeling. He never actually had full intercourse with me. Well, I don't think he did. No, I'm sure he didn't. I don't even know what happened after that.

As the interview went on, it became clear that somewhere along the line Victoria had chosen not to remember what had happened to her. Her sister Tess intimated as much to me during the interview. Victoria couldn't really state clearly exactly what had happened and Tess believed that she had chosen not to remember it all clearly. Victoria defended this position by saying that it was good that she didn't remember everything.

Because I can't remember it, I'm okay. If I don't remember it, it can't upset me [laughs]. I'm very practical [laughs]. I feel a bit cheated. Not cheated; I feel like there must be something wrong with me. There's women that are still devastated like 20 years after it happened. And I feel like, I'm quite happily going. To me, it happened. There's nothing you can do. It's happened. Stuff like this happens in life. You've survived, you're okay.

Just as many other children do, Victoria blamed herself for what happened to her and believed that she should have been able to stop it from happening.

> I feel guilty. I suppose another reason I never told anybody, or too many people, is that I felt that I was to blame, because I was 16 and older when stuff like this was going on and I thought that, at that age, a 16 year old ought to be able to say, 'Fuck off and leave me alone', or, you know, get out of the situation, like run away from home. But it never occurred to me to run away from home. I just stayed and put up with it.

Victoria's biggest fear was that history would repeat itself. She was obviously worried that her new boyfriend might sexually abuse her daughter but felt totally unable to talk to him about her fears, in case he became angry with her. I was concerned that she seemed frightened to broach the subject with him and to put clear boundaries in place for her own daughter.

> My biggest thing is, like I said, I've found a partner, and we'll probably get married and he's going to be a stepfather. And my biggest thing is leaving my daughter alone with him. I can't help it, and I'm terrified it's going to ruin the relationship. He's going to eventually cotton on one day that I won't leave her alone with him, and I'm terrified of telling him 'I won't leave you alone' because you're supposed to trust them. But I can't. I'm terrified that, what if I go along and make the same mistake?'

Victoria's experiences were extremely confusing for her, mainly because of her mother's collusion with her stepfather. She felt ashamed that she had been unable to stop the abuse when she was 16. She remained frightened of her mother, who had manipulated her for most of her life. But she also remained stoical and determined that these experiences had not affected her badly, while worrying that she was somehow vulnerable to repeating history with her own daughter and her new fiancé. Her sister Tess thought that she didn't remember everything and was in denial to a certain extent. I must admit that I wondered about that, too, but Victoria insisted that her pragmatic approach helped her to get on with her life.

Victoria's successful avoidant coping

Similarly to Bert, Victoria used avoidant coping as a survival strategy to some considerable apparent success. She was able to put the events of her childhood out of her mind and not dwell on them. This proved a highly successful coping strategy for her, which had helped her to move on with her life. This type of avoidant coping strategy is often used by people who have experienced more severe abuse and is, therefore, more likely to be linked with poorer outcomes in adult life.[1] However, many women claim that their use of denial and suppression has been beneficial for them, contrary to these findings.[2] Refusing to dwell on experiences and positively reframing them have been used as coping strategies among more well-adjusted groups of child sexual abuse survivors.[3]

I probably gained more of a sense of the possible level of avoidant coping used by Victoria because I interviewed her with her sister. Before Tess arrived, Victoria told me that there were some parts of her story that she hadn't yet told Tess. And Tess' body language told me that she thought that Victoria was failing to remember much of what had happened to her. But the result was that Victoria seemed calmer and more accepting of her childhood than Tess and less distressed by past events. It has been suggested that there is a continuum in terms of the ways in which women escape as children, from conscious and voluntary methods like daydreaming or concentrating on other pleasurable activities to unconscious and involuntary methods such as dissociation or repression of memories.[4] Perhaps conscious avoidance is functional and unconscious avoidance or dissociation is less so. This strategy certainly seemed to work for many years for Angelo.

Angelo's story – 'my wife's an angel'

Angelo was an attractive man in his late fifties. He had been brought up as an Italian migrant in Australia. His father had been interned for three years during the Second World War. During that time Angelo had formed a close bond with his mother. As a young boy Angelo was sexually stimulated by an employee and a female customer at his parents' shop. He didn't tell anyone about these incidents.

Angelo went on to become a successful businessman, get married and adopt children. He believed for many years that his sexual experiences with women had not affected him. However, after getting married, he was unable to have sexual intercourse with his wife. Instead he had a series of sexual encounters or affairs with married women. When his first marriage collapsed, he remarried and the same thing happened all over again.

Recently, Angelo had become quite depressed and suicidal and had talked to a psychiatrist about his problem with intimacy. He seemed to be severely depressed at the time of the interview. He didn't believe that his particular problem could be solved by anyone. He seemed to be thinking things through during the interview and to be making new connections between his childhood sexual experiences, his ongoing problems with sexual intimacy and his suicidal feelings. This is Angelo's story.

> Well, my little story starts back when I was 11 years of age. My mum and dad were Italian migrants and we had a shop and employees. And the most, clearest impression that I've got of what happened was that this lady, who was

probably my mother's age from memory, would take me up the stairs to the landing, which led up into the rooms. And she would, by memory, she would fondle me and do things. And this again from a child's memory, it's not my own memory, went on for a long time. I didn't really know, I didn't tell my parents. I've told nobody.

And then there was also another lady, a customer. My mum would ask me to deliver to her house in the afternoons. She would always have some kind of a cowboy or Indian present for me, toy leathers and cap guns, and she would take all my clothes off and put these leathers on with little cap guns. Or it would be no clothes on but just a thing round my head with a feather, and a little Indian kind of vest. And it never bothered me in the sense that I became mentally affected.

Throughout the interview, Angelo insisted that he hadn't been affected by these childhood experiences while at the same time describing how he had been influenced. He never defined his experiences as sexually abusive. The idea of a woman committing a sexual assault on a young boy tends to confront our assumptions about masculinity and femininity and may make a young boy like Angelo feel a sense of humiliation and betrayal at being abused by a woman who is supposed to be a nurturer and caregiver.[5] This may have been complicated further by the fact that Angelo idealised his mother and had a poor attachment to his father.

I loved my mother but I didn't love my father the way I loved my mother. My father being an Italian was interned during the war, and that was when I was born, and I spent the first three years of my life with my mother. Now my father's appeared and I never liked the idea of this man, so I've never really accepted him as being my father in a sense.

I've never had trouble with women; women are just attracted to me. I like women and women like me. Then I met this girl. We didn't have sex, we just got close. And then she just left her husband. We were married overseas, came home married. That was a great relationship, we were married for 20 years, terrific, but the sex was terrible. She couldn't have children. The real reason why she didn't get pregnant was we never really had sex. We ended up adopting the most beautiful children. And I could never have sex with her because she reminded me of my sister. So I did the usual thing, the animal that I was, I had sex with everybody. Anybody but her, but we were very close. I can almost remember every single one, and there was a lot of them, probably over a hundred. But there was something wrong about it. In the end we separated.

I was surprised and saddened when Angelo described the sexual difficulties that he had in his first marriage. He seemed to be able to have sexual intercourse only with women that were unattainable, i.e. those married to someone else but available for one-night stands with him. I started to wonder whether or not he actually despised women.

> With my second wife, we haven't had sex for two and a half years. I've been to the doctor's, I've done all that crap. Nothing works. Viagra doesn't work. I've had injections into the penis, that doesn't work. What's wrong is that there's no feeling in my mind to have sex. And she's so loving; this woman is just so bloody special. She's like an angel. And I don't know why God's given me a second chance.
>
> As soon as I love the woman, have deep feelings for her, I can't have sex with her. I feel that they're either my mother or my sister. I can't have sex with them. The women that I've had relationships with, there's the element of danger and, without being disrespectful to women, it's treating women like sluts. Terrific sex, but I would never want to go and see them again. What's worrying me now is that I'm looking at younger girls.

I felt uncomfortable when Angelo hinted that he was becoming attracted to younger women as he grew older. The sad thing was that he found it difficult to seek help because he knew that it was taboo to talk about being sexually abused by a woman. Growing up a Catholic, he may have experienced an additional cultural barrier just as American women with Hispanic backgrounds find disclosure difficult because of the high value placed on virginity within their culture.[6] But he was mainly worried that other men would dismiss his experiences as not really abusive, because he had been sexually abused by women.

> You can't talk to Italian parents about sexual things. No, you can't do that. Who else was there to talk to? You can't talk to male friends, because they'd say you're bullshitting, or you're lucky, or you hit the lottery. So who are you going to talk to? They say go to a doctor. That's bullshit; you can't go to a doctor and talk. You're not going to talk to a Catholic priest, for God's sake. I can't talk to males. If I told this to a male he'd say, 'You ought to be so lucky.' Men think that that's great.
>
> I would like just to go to sleep. I'm a coward, I'm just a bum. I despise myself. I wish I had the guts to end it, because there's no point. I have no manhood. I have nothing. And people see me and they go 'You're okay, everything's fine,' but inside I'm not a man. If a man can't feel he has a life and can't have sex with his wife. These are good women and you don't penetrate good women. That's the fucking problem. How do you get out of that? You can't.

There was an obvious contradiction in Angelo's story. He described how his childhood sexual experiences had not impacted on his life. At the same time he described his ongoing sexual difficulties and his suicidal feelings, which he was beginning to see as connected to these experiences. Angelo seemed to be re-storying his life during the interview. His distress was palpable.

Angelo divided women in a stereotypical way into 'angels' and 'sluts'. Angels were good women like his mother, his sister and his two wives. The sluts were married women who wanted to have sex with him. These were the only women he was able to have sex with and he did so in a compulsive manner. He was proud of his reputation as a 'Ferrari' not a 'Volkswagen' in terms of his sexual conquests. However, this image of himself no longer completely satisfied him. As a man in his fifties, he simply wanted to be able to have a normal sex life with his second wife. He was also concerned about his attraction towards young women, having had sexual encounters with women of all ages 'from 70 to basically 16'.

Minimisation of Angelo's sexual abuse by women

Feminists have argued that men are not treated as if they are damaged goods when abused in the same way that women are. Instead they tend to be seen as adventurous,[7] especially young boys who have sexual intercourse with older women. It seems to me that this makes things even more difficult for them. The experience of young boys such as Angelo is minimised by a society that does not view women as victimisers or young boys as suffering as a result of sexual activity with older women.[8] The idea of a female victimiser goes against feminist theories of child sexual abuse, based on ideas of power, control and patriarchy.[9] This makes it very difficult for men to disclose heterosexual experiences.

These gender issues are also reflected in the type of therapy that men give and receive compared to women. As was the case for Angelo, men are less likely than women to receive abuse-focused therapy after disclosing child abuse, and male clinicians are less likely than female clinicians to give abuse-focused therapy.[10] In one study only two out of 42 men who had been sexually abused received related treatment, even though they had all attended counselling.[11] Certainly, Angelo had seen his local doctor and a psychiatrist but was still feeling the need to talk to someone about his problems, which he saw as impossible to resolve.

I was concerned about Angelo after the interview and phoned to check on his well-being. He had found the conversation useful and had felt very relieved to be able to talk openly about his experience. I found our conversation challenging, partly because it was hard to hear about a young boy being sexually abused by a woman and partly because he was obviously in such a lot of psychological pain at the time of the interview. Similarly, my interview with Jim had a big impact on me and makes disturbing reading.

Jim's story – 'I just moved on'

Jim, also in his fifties, was tall and lanky with a deep gravely voice. He came from a relatively poor, single-parent home. He went to boarding school at 13, where he was digitally penetrated, caned and then anally penetrated by a master for nearly two years. Jim found this whole experience terrifying. He felt deeply ashamed about what had happened and the interview was the first time he had spoken to anyone about his experiences.

As an adolescent Jim met two people who helped him enormously. One was a young girl with whom he had an enjoyable heterosexual relationship. This brief relationship gave him an enjoyable experience of love and affection, leading to sexual desire, and helped him to feel like a normal, heterosexual male. The other person was a tradesman who took him under his wing and became his mentor. Jim used to watch him work and eventually became his apprentice.

Jim led the roving life of a bushman for many years, moving from town to town looking for work. As an adult he became involved with women who enjoyed bondage and discipline (B&D), with whom he was able to re-enact his childhood sexual experiences, playing both roles. He felt a great deal of shame just describing this behaviour.

> I suppose it started when I was 13. I came from a sort of an odd background. My mother was a pretty good woman, pretty hard-working woman. She came into money and she sent me to a school. There was a school teacher there. He seemed to take a particular liking to me. He used to say that he was going to 'try to help me to develop into a better adult'. The first time I had to attend his office for discipline, he told me to take off my shorts, my jocks, bend over his desk. He placed his hand in the middle of my back, and stuck a finger up my bum I suppose is the only way I can describe it, which was very greasy, and very frightening, and scared hell out of me. He then caned me, told me to put my shorts on and go.
>
> This happened on probably, I don't know, two more occasions similar to that, maybe three times. By then I was over the shock of it. My biggest fear I think was discovery, to be quite honest. The next time, the same thing, bend over the desk, he fingered me. He then caned me and told me to stay there. He rubbed my buttocks. And there was a window and I used to watch him in the reflection. While he was massaging my buttocks I could see that he had his penis out and erect. And I thought, 'There's no way he's going to put that in there.' I just went cold. And that was more of less how it happened sort of throughout my fourteenth year, into my fifteenth year.

As Jim told me his story, I sensed his acute sense of shame about what had happened to him at the hands of this man. He avoided eye contact with me for the first half of the interview, choosing to look at the floor instead. I was shocked, not so much by his story, but by the way he had internalised this intense feeling of shame.

> I could never tell anyone because I was embarrassed, ashamed, and I couldn't get a sort of a grip of it, because you lived with the idea in those days that teachers, they did no wrong. I never, ever told anyone about it. And then just one day, he wasn't there any more. He left, and I don't know what became of him. I did hear that he joined some sort of religious sect. I'm sure he wasn't doing it to anyone else, what he was doing to me. Why he had me isolated I don't know. I sometimes think it was because of my background. He punted that I wouldn't say anything at home.

Not only was Jim ashamed of what had happened to him but he also felt ashamed that he had somehow been chosen by this teacher, perhaps because of his poor background. But Jim was a battler and had a great capacity to see the good in people and in situations. His parting comment to me was that 'self-pity is the worst bloody disease that you can have'. He described two individuals from his school days that had really helped him to overcome his experiences.

> During that period there was a girl that worked in the kitchen. We used to meet in the park, and that led on to a boy–girl relationship of a normal type. We did all the normal things, or things that I've learnt to be normal as I've gone through life. And I think those few months probably bloody hauled me back from the edge of being a complete zombie. I was very distrusting of people. There'd be no way I'd be sitting here talking to you, if I hadn't had that. She taught me to trust people. Not long after she turned 18, she disappeared. But that period, I think, was the saving of me mentally; otherwise I think I would have been a complete crackpot. And I've had reasonably normal relationships with girls since. I've had some bloody odd ones too.
>
> There was a man who worked with animals. He said, 'I'll teach you a trade.' I spent two years in his shadow. I was always on the duck, I was just nervous of people, new people I couldn't handle. I'm still a bit like that, I still seek reclusive work: I worked with animals for a long time. I've sort of worked in isolated places. I did marry. It was a bloody disaster. I was a rodeo rider for a long time, back in the days when there used to be travelling boxing troupes. But no, I didn't bury meself [sic] in drugs and grog and self-pity, I just moved on with life. I couldn't see any reason to feel sorry for myself.

Recently, Jim had started to reconsider what had happened to him as a child. He recognised the severity of his experiences and the impact that they had on his sex life in particular.

Later on, when these sort of things started to get on the news and the word paedophile appeared and suddenly the local bloody scoutmaster's in all sorts of trouble, or the bloody Baptist minister. That actually amused me to a certain extent. I thought, 'I wonder how bad these people have been.' I lived with what I consider a bloody monster.

Jim had started to recognised that his involvement in B&D had been stimulated by his experiences at school and this disturbed him. Occasionally, he threw out comments to check whether or not I was sitting in judgement of him, such as: 'You're probably absolutely, bloody disgusted? And think "Jesus, what a bastard of a fellow that is," which I wouldn't blame you for one minute if you did.' I tried to reassure him with my body language and tone of voice that I was not disgusted by his behaviour as an adult. And, we both knew that, as a child, he didn't have a choice.

To a certain extent it did bloody affect me. When I was working in the city, I played with a bloody nurse and she'd bend over the desk, and I'd smack her bum with a cane and then we'd have sex. I sort of thought about my previous bloody show and then I thought, 'What I'm doing here is virtually the reverse of what used to happen to me as a bloody kid.' But she lapped it up, she loved it. At one period, I did think I should go and talk to somebody. Here I am [laughs] confessing it to you. I've never told bloody anyone.

Jim was humiliated and brutally treated by a sadistic teacher and yet he felt ashamed of what had happened to him. This subtle transfer of shame from the victimiser to the child seems to be such a destructive element of these narratives.

What I've realised is that I've never put it down, really. I think I've put it down, maybe when I say to you, 'No, I've moved on,' but it's always just been in the back of my bloody mind. At different times I've been involved with bloody women that like to have their bottom smacked. When I'm away from that, I bloody don't like myself at all, and that goes back to that period of my life, definitely. In some ways I think I'm probably hitting back. Probably in my subconscious I'm telling on him. I'm thinking, 'I'll bloody tell on you, you bastard.'

Like Bert, Jim showed great resilience in choosing not to dwell on the memory of what had happened to him at school. As he described the process of leaving the past behind him, he gestured with his hands to show the separation between his past and the new life he created. He chose to focus on the good times that he had with the girl. He knew that his relationship with her and with the tradesman had been very influential in helping him to get his life together. He chose to count his blessings and focus on these positive relationships, rather than dwell on the horror of his experiences at the hands of a sadistic teacher. I can only hope that Jim felt better after 'telling on him' and that his story will be useful to others in their struggle to move forward in their own lives.

Jim's feelings of shame and learned sexual behaviour

I shouldn't have been surprised when Jim expressed such intense feelings of shame about his childhood experiences, since many male victims of childhood sexual abuse experience shame and are more likely to do so than women. As a result, many men minimise their childhood sexual experiences. It is possible that some male victims develop problems with sexual dysfunction or sexual deviance, partly as a result of connecting sex and shame.[12] Concealing sexual abuse is one strategy that men frequently adopt to avoid being rejected or disbelieved and they are also more likely to employ strategies of avoidance or acceptance than women.[13]

Jim had recently started to recognise that he hadn't been able to leave it all behind, as he had once hoped. He felt ashamed and disturbed by his adult involvement with B&D. There was no suggestion that this activity involved children in any way, but Jim was clearly concerned that what he was doing was re-enacting his experiences at school. He showed great courage in coming forward to be interviewed and, when asked why he had done so, he admitted that he had finally decided to tell on this school master. He wanted to 'expose the bastard' who had frightened and humiliated him all those years ago. Like Jim, Peter had also kept his experiences a secret for a very long time.

Peter's story – 'it was exciting and fun'

Peter was an engineer in his late forties who had recently separated from his wife because he was having an affair. He was originally from a farming background. Whenever his family stayed with their city cousins, he was involved in sexual activity with a male cousin who was 15 years older than him. Peter thought that these events started when he was seven and stopped when he was 14. He found it exciting at the time.

Peter felt a certain amount of guilt and was also frightened of his father's response, if he ever found out. He chose to tell no one about his experiences until he got married. Peter believed that these experiences had no impact on him. He thought that he had put them behind him and moved on. However, recent publicity about paedophilia had unsettled him and had made him start to question his own beliefs.

Peter felt a certain frustration with the media coverage of childhood sexual abuse. He was in the process of reconsidering whether he had been more affected than he had earlier realised. In fact, he surprised himself by becoming quite tearful at one stage during the interview, when he spoke about his fears that other children might have suffered because he hadn't told anyone. This is how Peter described his experiences.

> I was the victim of paedophilia. The perpetrator was a male who was my cousin, but he was much older, probably 10 to 15 years older. And we used to visit the family. We lived in the country, and they lived in the city. He used to take advantage of me on those occasions. And he made me feel like it was normal. He would talk a lot about sex with me, in terms of male–female relationships, but it always ended up being a physical, homosexual relationship in which he was the controller of the situation. But he put it in such a way that I didn't feel that it was wrong. Oh, well, sorry, I suppose I knew. He used to say things like 'Don't tell your parents about this. *We* could get into a lot of trouble about this.'
>
> This may seem a bit strange but I was quite excited about it at times, because it was a sexual experience, so it was interesting and exciting for me. But it was always fairly one-sided. This went on for quite a number of years. I was afraid to tell anybody. I wasn't game to tell my parents. And I was frightened for myself as much as for what might happen in terms of aggravation in the family. So I kept it totally a secret.

Peter's story demonstrated how difficult it can be for children to tell anyone about what is happening to them. In general, disclosure rates are thought to be relatively low with 60–70% of adults choosing not to make a disclosure during childhood.[14] Disclosure is even less likely when the perpetrator is a family member,[15] as was the case for Peter. Like other children, Peter would have worried about his parents' likely response. 'Will they believe me or will they believe the denials of the other? Will they really do something to help me or will they punish me for having talked about it?'[16] Given Peter's close relationship with the victimiser, it would be harder for him to convince the family about what was happening to him.

> The last time was when I went to the city to a sporting carnival. At that stage I had more knowledge that this is not the right thing to do. And at that particular sports carnival I didn't do very well, and in my mind I put it down to the sexual act the night before. And I think that played on my mind. I still see him to this day, and every time I see him I react. I can see what's happened in the past but I've bottled all that inside. My parents are still alive, and I wouldn't want to create any hurt by raising the issue at this late stage of their lives. I haven't done anything about it. I got on with my life; it didn't seem to affect me.

Peter seemed to be surprised when he became tearful during our conversation because, up until that point, he had been telling himself that he had not been greatly affected by past events. He obviously felt guilty because he hadn't exposed his cousin and he was worried that other children might have also suffered as a result.

> So I basically got on with my life, and, you know, got married, four kids and that sort of thing. But as time went on, there was more and more public awareness of paedophilia, and especially with the problems with the churches and their boarding homes. And I thought, 'Should I have put this guy in?' Because I don't think I was the only, in fact I know I'm not the only person he approached. I'm not sure whether he actually assaulted anybody else. I've got no knowledge of that. I suspect he did. I'm sure I'm not the only victim, and as the awareness became more I thought, 'Well, maybe I've done the wrong thing in not raising this issue,' [with tears in his eyes] but I've continued to take that stance and I've only ever, you're the second person that I've ever spoken to about this. My wife's the only other person I've spoken to. I never, ever mentioned it to my male friends, never ever, and I wouldn't.

Peter seemed to be experiencing difficulties forming intimate and satisfying sexual relationships. This difficulty has been described by other men who have had sexually abusive experiences as children. Some avoid sexual activity altogether, some feel panic or terror when contemplating sexual activity, and some feel that they are performing sexually rather than engaging in an intimate act.[17] This last description seemed to fit for Peter.

> I relayed to my wife the story of my experience with paedophilia, and she said, 'Well, maybe the fact that there was no love in that relationship, it was purely a physical relationship, that I look on a relationship as physical rather than as a proper, loving relationship. And for that reason, sex is just a physical activity; it's not so much love. I don't focus on the love side of it.' And that may be why I'm happy to go off with another woman and have sex with her. And I think it's got a lot of credence actually.

Peter was willing to talk about the fact that he had found his early sexual experiences physically exciting and enjoyable. He admitted that he had tried to repeat his experiences with boys of his own age and was now relieved that they had shown little interest.

> I can still see the images of the times I was raped, but I didn't regard it as rape. And, as I said, there was perhaps this very strange thing: I thought it was exciting and fun. I was strongly heterosexual. I've never had any inclination towards homosexuality, and I know this is an enlightened era and we should have tolerance of homosexuals, but I have very little tolerance of them. Whether

that's also something that came out of this relationship or not, I don't know. I actually tried to carry out homosexual acts on some of my friends. Because you see I must have had this notion that it was normal to do this. And fortunately they reacted and said, 'No, I don't want to get involved,' which I'm very glad that they did, because that could have been very bad for me.

I was aware of Peter's struggle to come to terms with his decision to keep his sexual abuse secret, and his growing concern that he might have aided and abetted a paedophile by doing so. His motivation was to protect his family and this remained important to him as an adult.

One of the things I feel guilty about is whether I should have informed somebody. You know that's the thing that now probably gets at me the most. Has he abused somebody else, because I didn't spill the beans, you know? And has somebody been seriously hurt as a result of that? But my motivation was protecting my family, and Mum's family in particular. Whether that was right or not, I don't know. It was just a decision I made as a young teenager that I wasn't going to take it any further. I've always tried to protect people. And there's this thing about you're going to get in trouble with your parents. I mean I was petrified about not only what Dad would dish out to the other family, but what he'd dish out to me. He would probably have flown into a rage, and hopped into the car with a shotgun.

Like many others, Peter was starting to wonder about the impact of his experiences on his ability to sustain close relationships. Peter's wife believed that he saw sex as a physical, rather than as an intimate or relational, experience. He could relate to this explanation because his own parents had rarely showed any affection towards each other. He had a practical marriage and enjoyed a good sex life, but felt no strong bonds with his wife. He was not emotionally involved with the woman he was having an affair with either, and he admitted that their relationship was purely physical.

Peter's confusion over his physical arousal

Becoming aroused and experiencing pleasure complicates the experience of child sexual abuse for children of both genders. However, there is an added complication when a young boy became sexually aroused during an early sexual experience with a male, thereby raising concerns about homosexuality. If his body responds physiologically, there is a fear that the victimiser somehow knew that he would respond and had chosen the boy because of his hidden homosexuality.[18] Given that traditional masculinity is associated with compulsory heterosexuality, along with toughness and emotional restraint, a young boy who has become aroused during a homosexual experience is likely to feel a great deal of confusion and shame. This acts as a barrier to making a disclosure.

Peter found his sexual experiences with his older cousin interesting and exciting. Although he was homophobic and claimed to be 'strongly heterosexual', as an adolescent he tried to have 'penetrating [sic] sex' with boys of his own age at school. He saw this as experimental behaviour. The boys that he approached showed no interest in being involved and, as an adult, he seemed relieved by that. He thought that if his friends had been interested, things could have worked out badly for him. Although Peter saw masturbation sessions between boys as fairly normal, he saw his own sexual behaviour towards other boys as unusual. I thought that he showed great courage in taking about this issue.

NARRATIVE OF A SILENCE RECENTLY BROKEN

Looking for the common threads between these stories, I have termed this a *narrative of a silence recently broken*. This is a resilient narrative told by four men and women.

Initially, during the interviews, all four men and women described how their experiences had had no real impact on their lives. All had experienced some feelings of shame, self-blame and responsibility for what had happened to them. They felt that they should have been able to prevent events from occurring and feared the consequences of discovery. Since these events continued until they were in their mid-teens, their feelings of shame and self-blame grew over time. For Jim and Peter the shame increased when they realised that their experiences were homosexual in nature. This shame helps to explain why they chose a *narrative of a silence recently broken* for many years.

Feelings of shame seem to conflict with the assertion that their childhood sexual experiences had had no apparent ill effect on them. However, they reported being very successful at putting their thoughts and feelings to one side. They had learned how to move on with life, without dwelling on the past. Victoria, Angelo, Jim and Peter chose not to think about their experiences. They all demonstrated resilience by being able to lead normal lives, hold down satisfying jobs, get married and have children.

None of these men and women had talked to anyone about their experiences when they were children. However, the contradictory name of this narrative does not relate to a feeling of being silenced as children. Instead, it refers to their active choice to remain silent in adulthood. For Jim, it was the first time that he had told anyone, and the others had only told their intimate partners as adults. They all had slightly different reasons for not telling, from a belief that there was nothing to tell to fear of being punished in some way. There was a sense in which recent media coverage of child sexual abuse had made Peter feel bad about keeping his experiences a secret.

A *narrative of a silence recently broken* is a contradiction in terms and it is easy for the reader to project her or his own interpretations onto this silence. As you read these stories, you may have been thinking that their choice not to tell anyone was part of a pattern of denial and avoidance. This may be true, and such avoidant coping may well have been highly functional for them.

The reason that these men and women chose to break their silence at this particular point in time needs to be examined. The difficulties that they faced in their adult lives may have accumulated to such a point that they were re-examining the past to look for an explanation. Alternatively, the social context and media exposure around the issue of child sexual abuse may have prompted this reconsideration.

In recent years, Victoria and Peter had started to talk about their experiences using different language. Victoria talked about 'sexually molestering', and Peter described himself as a 'victim of paedophilia'. He assumed that paedophiles were homosexual. As Peter said:

> I've only used that word [rape] today because that is, in today's world, that's what it is. It was rape. I mean, well, I wasn't a consenting adult so that constitutes rape. And paedophilia, I mean, I suppose I would have just said he was a poofter in those days.

Contemporary societal views and media coverage of the topic of paedophilia appeared to have influenced particularly the men that I interviewed. They had begun to wonder whether or not their sex lives had been negatively influenced by what had happened to them. They had started to make possible connections between these experiences and the difficulties they had experienced in their intimate lives. In slightly different ways, Angelo, Jim and Peter were all questioning their ability to have fulfilling, intimate sexual relationships with women and their sense of self as loving, sexual partners.

Although most of the men and women that I interviewed felt that they were the least likely people to become victimisers because of what they themselves had been through, Angelo, Jim and Peter all admitted to being concerned about some aspect of their sexual behaviour as adults. They admitted that the line between normal and deviant sex would have been fairly easy for them to cross. But they all reported that they had not crossed this line.

However, it is important to acknowledge that men are still far more likely than women to move from being victims to becoming victimisers, particularly those who have been sexually abused by a female relative.[19] This move often happens relatively young, before the boy has reached the age of 14. By this age, some young boys will be sexually abusing other children. Clearly, there is a need for a great deal more research to explain the complicated dynamics which lead some men and women to continue sexual abuse into the next generation.

This only happens in a minority of cases and there is not a one-to-one relationship between child sexual abuse and becoming a perpetrator of child sexual abuse.

In trying to understand why these men and women had maintained silence at least until very recently, it is useful to look for differences between this group and others described in this book. For most of them, their sexual experiences began when they were adolescents rather than young children and, therefore, did not last as long. They didn't start at a very young age or at a developmental stage when they were even more vulnerable. Two had sexual experiences with people they knew, rather than with members of their own family. Overall they experienced less child maltreatment at home, had relatively good relationships with their parents and their peers, were able to find satisfying work as young adults and avoided drug and alcohol dependence. They had not sought help and only Victoria had attended more than two sessions of therapy. In other words, they came from relatively well functioning family environments.

In the following chapter, another narrative shared by five men and women will be described. This is a very different narrative experienced by those who felt that their childhood sexual experiences had a major impact on them and continued to affect them as adults. More than most, these men and women were still in the process of working through their experiences and trying to make sense of them. Their ongoing suffering is apparent in their stories.

SUMMARY

Key points

- The narratives told by these four men and women challenge the idea that all people who have childhood sexual experiences with adults believe that they have been badly affected by them.
- These men and women told socially unacceptable narratives of not being severely impacted by their experiences.
- Apart from Victoria, they grew up in relatively well functioning families compared to other people that you will meet in this book. They were not physically or emotionally abused at home and were slightly older when these events took place. This may have helped them to find the resilience not to dwell on their experiences and to move on with their lives.
- However, they still felt a measure of shame and self-blame about what had happened and had recently started to be concerned about the long-term impact of their childhood experiences on their intimate relationships and on their sexual behaviour as adults.
- This seems to be the reason that this is a *narrative of a silence recently*

broken. These men and women chose silence in childhood. However, they
had eventually found a language and had chosen to speak up as adults –
at least to their partners, although not necessarily to other family
members.

- Some, like Peter, felt pressured by recent media coverage of child sexual
abuse and paedophilia. They felt guilty that they had not spoken out about
their experiences, in order to protect other children from harm.
- It is important to consider whether or not to take these narratives at face
value or to see these men and women as in denial.
- It is possible that their ability to suppress thoughts about their childhood
sexual experiences for many years may have operated as a functional form of
avoidant coping, rather than as repression or denial.

CHAPTER 5

The need to remember and the need to forget

INTRODUCTION

Chapter aims
- Tell the narratives of five men and women who had painful memories of their childhood sexual experiences.
- Explore *the need to remember and the need to forget*.
- Describe the profound effect that their experiences had on them.
- Illustrate their need to forget and how they repressed their thoughts or memories.
- Examine their need to remember to make sense of their lives.
- Discuss this narrative in relation to the victim discourse.

This chapter explores the struggle that five men and women had between their need to remember what happened to them as children and their need to forget these painful memories. These are the problem-saturated narratives of victims who experienced ongoing suffering. These narratives are frequently found in the child sexual abuse literature, and are particularly common in the recovered memory literature. These men and women described their suffering as a result of traumatic childhood sexual experiences. They believed that these experiences had had a profound impact on them as children, and as adults. As Colin said, 'I just get to suffer this on my own.'

Among those who were affected traumatically, two main storylines emerged. The first was told by three people who had either recently recovered memories of incestuous childhood experiences or had come to recognise that their experiences had been incestuous. With the benefit of hindsight, they were starting to make sense of the difficulties that they had experienced during their lives. They were still in the process of remembering exactly what had happened and trying to accommodate this new information about themselves and their family members. As a result of this turmoil, they had a fragile sense of who they really were as people.

The second storyline was told by a man and a woman who had also been severely affected by their experiences. They had sexual contact mainly with non-family members, starting when they were as young as four years old. They were concerned about others whose lives were being ruined and, for that reason, wanted to remember more than they wanted to forget.

All five were still struggling with the impact of their childhood experiences and were too angry to move on with their lives. They felt that they had been damaged, violated and betrayed. Some felt that no one really cared about their suffering and that society had somehow let them down. They wanted to take part in the study in order to help other people avoid the pain and distress that they themselves had experienced.

There may be a developmental process involved in the evolution of these narratives. People may gradually move from one narrative to another. For example, some might have told *narratives of a silence recently broken* when they were younger, as a result of having blocked out all memories of events of their childhood. It is also possible that those currently telling *narratives of a silence recently broken* will go on to tell other narratives in later life.

SEARCHING FOR A SENSE OF SELF

Sylvia, Tess and Leo described how their incestuous experiences had not only had a huge impact on their lives, but helped to explain and make sense of their lives. Sylvia and Leo had both recently remembered these experiences during therapy. Sylvia felt intense anger, Tess felt confused and Leo felt great shame. Each had pushed aside or forgotten exactly what had happened to them. It was only as adults that they had remembered or realised that their experiences had been incestuous. This process helped to explain some of the difficulties that they experienced in their adult lives and to make sense of certain events. However, they experienced a sense of unravelling during the process.

Sylvia's story – 'raped by my father'

Sylvia was a woman in her late thirties, with a partner and a young son, living in a rural area. She described being brought up in a small housing commission home by a caring mother and an alcoholic father, in difficult economic circumstances. Her father had served in the army and ruled the family by fear. She described him as physically and emotionally abusive. It became clear that Sylvia was terrified of her father.

Eight weeks before the interview Sylvia had remembered being raped by her father at the age of eight. She cried as she told her story, tears of sadness and anger. This was a very raw interview and she used the word 'rape' over 30 times, repeatedly naming what he had done. Sylvia was in the process of changing her ideas about her upbringing as she tried to make sense of it. It helped to explain her emotional breakdowns, which she now preferred to call 'spiritual awakenings'. She appeared to be rewriting her own history in the room while talking about the rape by her father.

As she tells her story, you will see how Sylvia switches between anger and distress. She was suffering profoundly as she attempted to understand her father's inexcusable behaviour. As with many other stories in this book, you may find it painful to read. I certainly found it difficult to hear at the time.

> I found out that I had been raped by my father eight weeks ago. And before that point, I always felt that there was something wrong, something was undermining me. I felt I couldn't get what I wanted, what other people had, just normal things like a job, somewhere to live that's okay, you know. I've lived with the fact my father was an alcoholic. I've lived with the fact that he used to take pills. I've lived with the fact that we were constantly verbally abused, emotionally abused. We were yelled and screamed at, when he would come home from the pub. One of the memories is all of us children, and Mum included, sitting on the green lounge, some time of night with a bare bulb, and Dad is yelling and screaming at us six kids and Mum. And he's overbearing, and I come out of my body, and I see it from above, from up in the roof. They're all just crying. And I would have been three, four, five.
>
> So all this time I thought that I was a product of an alcoholic. We were brought up, fucking commissioner places, on the edges of town. We had bushland around us, bushland in front of us, kids in the neighbourhood, but it was fear-based fucking bullshit you know. Poor bastards we were, but we were alright, we were kids, we got through it.

I was struck by the harsh childhood that Sylvia described, in many ways similar to that of other children in this book. She not only experienced childhood sexual abuse, but also lived with a physically and emotionally abusive father, prone to drunken rages. This was another family of 'poor bastards'. It was hardly surprising that she struggled to create a good life for herself as a young woman, taking drugs, suffering from bouts of depression, and having more than one termination.

> In my twenties I was taking a few drugs. I never really wanted to; I'm not a person that takes drugs. I had the emotional breakdown. My brother and his wife looked after me. And they somehow pulled me through that emotional breakdown, major depression. I thought it was due to terminations that I'd

had, but now I realise that underlying that was this rape, done by my father to me. Unbelievable.

When I was getting better, I met John. I still had this outer shell of love and happiness, and I had a job and I was doing clay work, and singing, and dancing and playing drums, everything on the outside, the outside shell. The inside was this mash, this huge deep, dark hole [crying]. I wanted a family; I wanted to be a normal woman. I want a lover, a partner, someone I can trust myself as well, a job, a child, more children, a house, a property, llamas, alpacas, I want to live and move and create like others can.

During the interview, I was aware that Sylvia was hearing her own story and putting together the pieces of the jigsaw puzzle. She was beginning to realise all of the repercussions of her father's violence towards her and her siblings.

I lived with this monster for 17 years. I was raped by this monster. I was, and my brothers and sisters, and my mother were just demonised by this person. My other brother actually has the brains, but he was also annihilated by Dad. He would be sat on the lounge naked at night, and Dad would yell at him and scream at him while drinking beer and popping fucking tablets. Dad always used to accuse the boys of being drug addicts. Now all this time I wondered how come the boys would get picked on, but I never got picked on. But I'd already been raped, he's done the deed. He'd already annihilated me.

As a child, Sylvia had repressed all memories of what had happened to her, but as an adult she chose to tell her mother. She used powerfully emotive language to describe how her base chakra had been 'penetrated'.

I had to tell Mum, I wanted to tell her, but she didn't want to believe it. After I told her, and she accepted it, she went into a plummet. Guilt, hurt, fear, anger, and she was useless to me. Every step is not easy. Any decision takes so much working out, because there's no trust. My father abused me. He betrayed me. He turned me inside out, he fed me with fear, so how could I trust anything else, because I had been just raped; the life had been raped out of me. My base chakra had been penetrated and been annihilated from Mother Earth.

It was hard to interview Sylvia because she had recovered memories of being raped by her father so recently and her emotions were still very raw. She felt angry and betrayed, not only by her father, but by her mother and her older siblings who should have been able to protect her from her father.

Mum told me that she remembers him coming out of my room. And she also remembers seeing blood on the sheets. He berated me apparently before, and I was so scared and so frightened that I probably allowed it to happen too. Well, it happened, I didn't allow it, but I was forced into that corner. And when I'm with my therapist, I'm on that bed and I know he came from behind, and he did that to me, and my head was bumping up against a fucking wall. It's just full on, it is so full on [tearfully], it is so massive that there is no way that those fucking bastards can realise what they have done to a little girl, to thousands of millions of little girls.

I'm angry with Dad. What a fucking dickhead. And I'm angry at my Mum and my sister for not protecting me. I'm angry at my oldest brother, where was he? He was the oldest and he wasn't there. And because they didn't protect me I actually feel like they were part of the perpetration. I had a dream the other night that my brother also sort of raped me. But there's no way he did. But him not protecting me is equivalent to that happening.

Sylvia interprets her dream of being raped by her brother as a metaphor for what he did by failing to protect her against her father. Throughout the interview I could sense her struggling to work out what to believe and what not to believe. She didn't really want to believe that her father had raped her, let alone that her mother somehow knew what was happening. This dilemma is very common when people recover lost memories. She was extremely angry with her father who had destroyed her confidence and her potential, leaving her feeling empty inside. However, she was determined to overcome this and she was fighting hard to live in a way that transcended her childhood maltreatment.

Today I can see talents in me, I can see the intelligence, I can see the determination, I can see the confidence even though it's been shattered and annihilated, there's something there. There's an essence there. And I can see that by doing what he did, he killed that. He destroyed any hope I had of actually being an amazingly beautiful daughter and person. I couldn't feel on the inside of me, I could not feel anything except the heavy dread of living. And even though I'd try and I'd try, and I'm so damned determined to live this life, I had no real strength. It took every ounce of my energy just to establish myself as me, and I had to rebel, and push, and fight everything just to have a little corner of myself.

Sylvia's struggle with recovered memories

During the 1980s and 1990s, feminists argued that defining women as victims further stigmatised them and ignored the gendered social context of the crime. As a result, the terminology changed from victim to survivor in order to empower women. This semantic change may have made it possible for some women to move from being silent victims to being more vocal survivors.[1] Certainly some women have described embracing the identity as a survivor of child sexual abuse as helpful in providing them with a sense of solidarity with other women who have been traumatised as children.[2] Although Sylvia was very early in the process of recovering memories of childhood abuse, she was already showing signs of feeling some solidarity with other children who had been maltreated. She was also able to see herself as a survivor with strengths and sensible adaptive behaviours, rather than remaining stuck in the victim paradigm. It is possible that she will gradually move from telling a narrative of victimhood to a more optimistic survivor narrative in the future.

Tess' story – 'the abuse with no name'

Tess, Victoria's sister, was in her early thirties, lived in a rural town, and was married with young children. The sisters grew up in a highly sexualised environment. As an adolescent, Tess was in the room when her mother and stepfather were having sex. During these incidents, her stepfather would touch her sexually. After a failed attempt with Victoria, her stepfather had sexual intercourse with Tess from the ages of 14 to 16. This ended when Tess' mother, stepfather and sister Victoria moved to Australia, leaving Tess to live with her biological father overseas.

Tess described her stepfather as a gentle and loving man, who wanted her to keep things secret from Tess' mother. As an adult Tess moved to Australia and chose to remain friendly with her stepfather until he died. She had only recently begun to talk about these experiences with Victoria. She had started to agree with Victoria that they had been sexually abused. But she remained very confused about her mother's part in it all, especially because her mother knew exactly what was happening and had condoned it. Interestingly, neither sister named their mother as abusive despite her extreme behaviour towards them which started when they were very young.

> I do remember being tied to the bed one night by Mum, and Victoria the same night, because we'd had beds in the same room, and I had gloves on my hands. I think Victoria did too. And we were tied our hands up to the headboards, because Mum was going to have one night where I didn't suck my thumb and Victoria didn't pluck her eyelashes. She doesn't [looking towards her sister], she doesn't remember anything.

This was one of the themes running through this interview. Tess intimated several times that Victoria didn't really remember what had happened to her as a child. And yet Tess had only come to certain realisations herself when Victoria had started to name her own experiences as abusive. I was shocked when she described the way in which her mother had encouraged her stepfather to take her virginity.

> My stepfather [Jon] had a flat actually in the car park of the pub where they used

to drink, and we used to go there and in the flat was a queen-sized water bed, a television, a bathroom, that was about it. And they'd trot off to the pub, and they'd come home. And they'd have sex, right beside me. Jon used to actually touch me a lot while he was having sex with Mum and all that sort of stuff. She knew, because she used to tell me quite often that it was my fault. He was only supposed to help me lose my virginity and then he was supposed to stop after he took my virginity, he was supposed to stop. But he never did and Mum kept saying it was because I was throwing myself at him. A lot of the times Dad was at home, later on, and when they were going to the pub and I didn't want to go, [whispers] I hated Dad for that. I hated Dad for that so much.

It was fascinating to see how Tess and her sister Victoria had different recollections of their childhood. Whereas Victoria coped by refusing to think about things, Tess was still struggling to make sense of her childhood. She found it hard to cope with the complexity of her emotional response. She hated both her mother and her father for betraying her, but continued to feel loving towards her victimiser. She didn't understand why her mother had behaved in the way she did. When her mother had accused her of encouraging her stepfather, she accepted the blame readily.

Jon was so protective and so loving. That sounds really terrible to say about that man, but he was so loving and protective of us. But also in a sexual way. He was never violent. I mean, when we had intercourse it was always gentle and loving. He used to tell me how much he loved me, and I mean I was 14. And he used to say to me, 'I want to take you to Australia and we can have 10 kids and we can start our life together, because I've never met anyone I'm in love with so much as you. And we can't tell your mother that we're going.'

I can remember being totally frightened all the time. This is why my nerves are shot now, I'm sure of it. I am so jumpy. If anyone comes up behind me and I don't see them coming, I jump. For years, I spent, like if you were sitting on the couch, Mum would get up to empty the ashtray or something. There'd be a hand reach out, down your crutch. I was so aware that any second that Mum turned her back, there was going to be a hand somewhere on my body. I can remember being frightened. Jon never actually physically frightened me. Mum did.

The fact that her mother had condoned what had happened continued to confuse Tess. She was only just coming to terms with the idea that what had happened was abusive. She had begun to recognise her mother's behaviour as an act of betrayal but did not yet identify her stepfather as her abuser. Her experience was complicated by her experience of a loving relationship with her stepfather. As a result she still felt protective towards him, despite his behaviour.

> We were talking about it and Victoria said 'sexually molestering' and it wasn't until then that I put *me* in that category. What he did do was, he did sexually molest us, but I'd never put a name on it, I'd never thought. It wasn't until my sister told me that I'd actually been through it, that I realised, yes, that's what it was. But because it wasn't violence and he wasn't holding a knife to our throat and saying you know 'Shut up', or 'Don't tell your mother' or anything. Because to me, Mum knew. There's no way that she can be laying near me, having sex with a man, and not know that his hand is touching me.
>
> I knew it was wrong but I didn't know it was wrong. Like, to me, it shouldn't have happened but Mum said it should have happened, so that was okay because Mum knew about it. I don't think I've dealt with it. I mean I've never had counselling. The only person I've ever talked to about it is Victoria. But it is so frustrating because she doesn't remember a lot of it.

Tess had learned that overt sexual behaviour within families was normal and, as a result, she did not always demonstrate appropriate, self-protective boundaries. She explained that she was involved in sexual activities with older men as an adolescent, which she saw as a natural extension of being introduced to sex at a young age. She also described a situation in which she had been raped by her boyfriend and how she was more concerned about his self-inflicted injuries than her own physical and emotional pain. She was protective towards him, just as she was towards her stepfather.

> I was going out with this guy and he raped me and after it, he was so sorry that he'd done it that he punched this glass window and pulled back all the skin on his hand. And he went screaming out to the mates that were in the lounge room there. And I came out and I was hurting. He didn't rape me vaginally, it was anally. And I was hurting so much and I was bleeding from there, and I was so worried because he'd cut his hand. And I couldn't hate him either, yet I was screaming at him to stop, and he wouldn't stop.

It became clear that Tess knew that some of her reactions to events of the past weren't normal. She seemed to find the conversation useful and was trying to pluck up the courage to attend counselling. She also wanted to confront her mother about her betrayal of her daughters.

> I would really like to do some sort of counselling, but I've just always lost my nerve. I think they'd look at me and say, 'Well, what's wrong with you? You don't even hate him. This guy did this to you and you don't even hate him.' I want to confront her about this. I want to ask her why she let him do that. Was it because she was so in love with him? Which I don't believe for a minute. Or is it just because she's sick, you know? Why did she let all this happen? I hate

her so much, because to me this is all her fault. Even though she's not the one who had sexual intercourse with me, it was Jon, but I hate her for it. You know what I mean, and I hate her more now that I'm a mother, because I think, 'God, I could never do that to my kids.' I look at my kids and I just think, 'God I love them so much.' And I think, 'My mother can't have loved me. My mother, who gave birth to me, can't have loved me.'

The social construction of 'victims' like Tess

During the female socialisation process, young girls learn to suppress their 'masculine' emotions such as anger in order to remain in emotional connection with others. If they want to be seen as good women, they need to be passive and to suppress their wants and desires, and become the custodians of relationships.[3] It is ironic that women tend to silence their own thoughts and feelings, for the sake of maintaining relationships with others. Women and adolescent girls are often taught about their sexuality in relation to victimisation, disease and morality.[4] They are expected to 'contain' the sexual desire of adolescent boys and to take a moral stance on the issue of sexual intercourse, in order to be seen as good. If not, young women are often portrayed as sluts.[5] These socially constructed views influence the ways in which young girls respond to unwanted childhood sexual experiences and make them vulnerable to re-victimisation.

Tess was groomed by her stepfather, with her mother's consent, and became almost a willing victim. To this day she can't make sense of her feelings towards her stepfather or her mother. What happened to her was wrong and yet her mother seemed to think that it was alright. Growing up in such a confusing, sexualised home environment led her to experience further abusive sexual encounters in adolescence as part of a pattern of re-victimisation. She might have been labelled as a slut by others for behaving in this way. She had probably not come to grips with all of this at the time of the interview and needed to journey further, as did Leo.

Leo's story – 'a sweet innocent undamaged child'

Leo was a highly intelligent and sensitive man in his early fifties who was separated from his wife and children. The separation, coupled with his mother's death, had triggered a breakdown and a suicide attempt. He had moved to a small coastal town, was currently unemployed and attended counselling twice weekly. He had been diagnosed with dissociative identity disorder (DID) by a psychiatrist.

Leo was emotional during the interview as he described how his mother had sexually abused him as a child. He had disturbing memories of sexual contact with a group of young men, and a number of other incidents during adolescence. As a young man, Leo became a heroin addict, drank alcohol to excess and had non-relational sexual intercourse with both men and women. Gradually, his life settled down, he became drug free and went on to achieve success in his career.

Since his recent breakdown, more memories of childhood abuse had surfaced. Leo believed that, at a young age, he had split into many different personalities or 'alters', in order to cope with the painful events of his childhood. He was frightened that one day he would remember a shameful act of ritual abuse, and moved from belief to disbelief about aspects of his own story. He longed to be a child, and described himself as a child trapped in a man's body. There was a sense in which he needed to withdraw from reality into what he perceived as the safety of childhood, in order to avoid overwhelming feelings of shame.

> Mum was a fanatical Catholic. Dad's a Holocaust survivor. He's suffered terribly from terror and the effects. He used to have terrible nightmares. So I guess the environment from a very early age was terror and massive guilt and shame. Mum had a thing about men, she hated men, and she used to say in front of us, all the time, that she hated Dad.
>
> But she liked me more than I think was appropriate, and she did everything for me. Mum's side of the abuse was like she owned everything, my mind, my body, my soul, my spirit, my thoughts, my emotions, everything. She didn't ask me how I felt, she told me how I felt. She didn't see who I was. She didn't know me in fact. We were so enmeshed that I had no idea who I was. But she liked touching my body and she used to bath me right up into my teens. I think it was a form of love, but the thing that used to worry me, she used to wash me. She used to really make sure that my genitals were very, very clean.

I was aware that Leo had attended therapy sessions over the years and had read books about dissociative identity disorder. As a result he tended to use the language of therapy to describe his experiences, such as his enmeshment with his mother and his fragmentation into multiple personalities or insiders, following an incident of ritual abuse.

> There were a number of perpetrators, one-off incidents. There was a friend of Mum's whose son was grooming me. I think I must have had 'victim' written all over my face, because people used to walk up to me in the streets, on a bus, and invite me back to their place. It used to happen all the time. I don't have a lot of memory as to what actually happened.
>
> Something happened, though, around the age of 12. I've only just started to remember in the last couple of weeks. But the memories are too strong and they explain so much. It was like an initiation ceremony. I think that they were much older boys, like they were in their late teens. And it involved killing,

there was a lot of blood involved. I don't know whether it was a person or an animal, and the blood was all over my genitals. These are just brief memory flashes.

I'm DID [dissociative identity disorder]. I've got twins that are seven, one's a boy, one's a girl. Our little dog got run over when I was about seven. I wasn't allowed to cry because 'boys don't cry'. The only way I could deal with it was to create a girl who was allowed to cry and then banish her. So a lot of my insiders are twins because I have the part that Mum wants to see, the part that complies to Mum's expectations, and then the one that carries all the horror and the pain. I create them and then I'll send them away.

Leo believed that he had a fragmented identity as a result of his childhood experiences. He saw dissociation as a way of keeping himself safe.

When I was in the height of my alcohol and drug addiction, I'd wake up with a whole lot of people and not know how I'd got there. That was quite scary at times. I mean being DID, God only knows, like I don't know how I'd got there, whether it was the alcohol or whether I'd actually split off or dissociated, stuffed if I know. The beauty of dissociation is that it keeps me totally safe and I've basically chosen safety over the risk.

Ever since he had started to remember his childhood sexual experiences, Leo had been plagued with an overwhelming feeling of shame. He lived in terror of uncovering an abusive act that he had been involved with. He believed that this shame was inescapable and that he could never be forgiven, despite not being able to remember what he had actually done. His creative solution to this dilemma was to live as if he was a child.

There's no point in believing in God because I'm going to go to hell anyway. I'm beyond redemption. And all these good Christians always turn round and say, 'God will obviously forgive you,' and I think, 'Maybe.' I have difficulty believing that because I'm so bad, the shame is so intense and so deep. And I don't even know what I did wrong.

I feel like a child who is very good at pretending to be an adult, but I'm not an adult. It's just too dangerous to be an adult, because if I admit that I'm an adult, then the bad things that happened to me at 12 really did happen. If I'm still a child, then they haven't happened, and they're not real and it's all made up.

Leo certainly had a childlike quality to him. Like Peter Pan, he didn't want to grow up because that would mean facing up to terrible events that happened to him at a young age. He seemed locked in a struggle for survival.

I shave most of my body every day, which is very long part of my ritual, but I have to do it. If I'm a little child then the shame is nowhere near as intense. The moment I start to consider any possibility that I'm an adult then I have to incorporate that massive shame, and it's huge, it's crippling. If I allow that shame in, I basically just sit in a chair and I don't move because it just cripples me totally.

I see children in a playground, and there's such an incredible sense of long-ing. And I don't even know what it is that I'm longing for. It's that innocence, they are undamaged. Like they've got something that I've lost. That's been stolen from me I guess. My whole life's about how can I be that child again. But I think I'm intelligent enough to recognise I'm not going to find what I'm looking for in another child.

Towards the end of the interview, Leo told me of his yearning to be a child. He saw children as innocent and undamaged and longed to be like them. As he spoke he constantly checked to see whether or not I understood what he was saying or was judging him negatively.

Deep shame leading to dissociation and fragmentation in Leo

Leo described dissociation as an invaluable coping mechanism that was keeping him alive. It stopped him from experiencing great pain and from the urges that he had to end his own life. He believed that he had shut down his feelings as a child. He also used a combination of drugs, alcohol and non-relational sexual experiences as coping mechanisms as a young man.

Leo believed that he had a fragmented identity and suffered from dissociat-ive identity disorder. He was in the process of identifying and getting to know his 'alters', with the aim of integrating them. He still felt that he needed these alternative personalities and preferred to experience life through their eyes. Leo had a strong yearning to be a 'sweet, innocent, undamaged child' rather than a man in his fifties. He had made the unusual decision to live as a child, in order to keep himself safe. He was working hard to recover and putting all his energy into this goal. This made him different from Hope and Colin who were less clear about the way forward.

CAMPAIGNING FOR OTHERS

Hope and Colin felt very angry about the events of their childhood which had a major impact on their lives and continued to ruin other people's lives. They were both brought up in families that would now be described as neglectful, and experienced sexual contact with adults outside the family from the age of four. In different ways, they both attributed to these experiences many of their prob-lems in adulthood, such as feeling suicidal, excessive use of drugs and alcohol and having non-committed sex. Hope, in particular, wanted to remember her experiences and expose paedophiles whenever possible. Colin wanted to be compensated for his experiences but struggled between wanting to remember and wanting to forget, wanting to tell and wanting to remain silent.

Hope's story – 'an interrupted childhood'

Hope was a single mother of three, in her early forties, living in a rural area. She had been to art school and had previously worked in the childcare industry. She described herself as an 'anti serial child rapist campaigner'. She was raped by a neighbour from the age of four to nine, after which she managed to stop it from happening. She had three children with two different fathers but had decided never to get married. Her own children had been sexually abused and this had become the focus of her life – to bring paedophiles to justice. She agreed to do the interview because she felt so passionately about the topic.

Hope came from a family of five children in which all three girls had been sexually assaulted by three different men. She believed that her mother had also been sexually abused and that these experiences had made her incapable of protecting her children. According to Hope, this left her mother vulnerable to being targeted by paedophiles.

Hope said very little about her own childhood sexual experiences or their impact on her. Actually, it wasn't always clear whether she was talking about her own experiences as a child, her experiences as a mother, or someone else's experiences. Perhaps this was her own way of distancing herself from what had happened. She was full of intense anger and hatred towards paedophiles and had a good understanding of child maltreatment as an intergenerational issue.

> When it first started happening I did tell my mother but she was a victim of serial child rape herself. I think that she was so traumatised, and hadn't dealt with it, that she couldn't deal with it. And I remember telling her that my vagina was sore, that I was bleeding, and her response would be 'Oh just put powder on it.' She couldn't deal with it. I told my mother repeatedly and I think I stopped trying when I was about six. She just didn't want to know. I was getting a very negative response. In her opinion I was masturbating too much. It was my fault that this was happening. If she had been the mother she thought she was, I wouldn't have been the raped child [with an edge to her voice] I ended up being. And having the problems that I have.
>
> I'm one of five children, two brothers and two sisters. A very unsupportive extended family, so my mother wasn't really coping at all. I think the last thing she needed was having to admit that she wasn't looking after her children well enough. Or she was being targeted by paedophiles, because she'd been left unprotected, protecting even more unprotected people. I was palmed off in the holidays. I was like a disposable child, which actually saved me,

because every time they got rid of me off to the relatives that stopped him from raping me.

I was struck by the expression 'a disposable child' and thought that it was sad that Hope had found refuge from sexual abuse whenever she was 'palmed off' by her parents to stay with relatives. She seemed to believe that she had been able to stop the rapes from happening herself. She went on to describe how she longed to be normal and to fit in at school.

> After I stopped him raping me, when I was nine, I kind of realised that I was in a really bad situation. And up until I was about 12, I created an alternative personality. I put that part of myself aside, like a holiday, and tried to become normal I suppose. I was aware that I wasn't developing normally. I think that people who've had interrupted childhoods are good at putting on facades, because we live in a world that not only clips the tall poppies, but they step on the bent stemmed ones too. I had a permanent boyfriend from the time I was 14. I knew that these very good-looking boys found me attractive. They always had money and cars. Much to their delight I was quite keen to have sex, because I thought that was expected. I didn't realise that very few girls were actually having sex at that age.

In many ways Hope was very knowledgeable about paedophiles and understood the ways in which they groomed their victims. She was also knowledgeable about the rape of young boys and its impact on them. She had obviously thought about the issue a great deal. And yet she also seemed to confuse homosexuality with paedophilia or to link the two inextricably, and to see paedophiles and conspiracies everywhere.

> As I've grown up I've realised that men say all sorts of things but they do not protect their children. They say they will. They never do. As soon as they're confronted with the truth, and particularly if it's somebody that they know or is a friend of theirs, then they go the opposite. They will attack the children. 'How dare you say that about him? He's a nice man. You must be lying.' Of course, that destroys the relationship between the child and his parent which was, from my observation, exactly what the paedophile wants, to isolate the child even more. Any man with a young girlfriend is a paedophile.
>
> Male rape's not something that you hear a lot about because it's more stigmatised than female rape or child rape. But they're definitely out there. And one of them attached himself to me. I didn't realise, I knew he was homosexual, but I didn't realise that he was a serial child rapist. And he eventually attacked my youngest boy when he was six. And that led to the Department of Community Services interview assessment and where we are today, struggling to get a court

order against someone who has already been confirmed by the Department as having sexually abused my son. And he's still a raging homosexual, although he's a closet queen now.

Anyway he ends up being the guy who rapes my son, who I can't even get a court order out against. I don't want to say it in the court house, or in front of the police, but that Magistrate's definitely a paedophile. There's no doubt about that, I can smell 'em. That's why I'm very good with childcare. I've worked in before and after school care, vacation care, I've used my art to teach the children. I do a lot of creative classes, and I can spot 'em. I can spot it; I mean you've just got to look for a man who's hovering near a bunch of kids.

Hope believed that she was the target of paedophiles because she was willing to tell the police whenever she encountered someone she believed was a child rapist. She believed that she was up against a 'serious, serial child rape network which is built into our government departments'. Not surprisingly, she found it extremely difficult to trust anyone.

I'm more targeted by paedophiles now, as an anti serial child rapist campaigner than I was as a child. I am, in their eyes, the enemy, because I am not afraid to tell their dirty secret. I am not afraid to recognise those who I feel are taking advantage of children.

The world's filled with fakes and the paedophiles are the biggest fakes of all, because they make out they're decent human beings, and they know inside their heart they're not. And that's why they all commit suicide, because they're just so cowardly and gutless, that they'll never ever, ever be able to resolve their issue, they know they're doomed.

Hope's fury with homosexuals, paedophiles and the system

Hope seemed to realise early on that her development was far from normal. She grew up feeling hatred for men in general, for homosexuals, and for paedophiles in particular. She was contemptuous of men who volunteered to work with children and equated paedophilia with homosexuality. She was applying for victim's compensation on behalf of her adult son who was a victim of child sexual abuse and she had recently tried, and failed, to take out a restraining order against her son's abuser. This exacerbated her anger with the system.

When I read what Hope had to say, I agreed with many of the points that she made. But the way that she spoke at the time of the interview made it hard for me to hear her wisdom. She was so full of anger and radiated a white heat, probably related to not being believed and being dismissed in the past. She found it difficult to trust me and didn't want to have any contact with me after the interview. As an adult, campaigning against paedophilia seemed to have become an integral part of Hope's identity, in a similar way to Colin.

Colin's story – 'society owes me'

Colin was in his early thirties, unemployed and living in a large country town with his partner and their four children, all from previous relationships. Colin had numerous sexual experiences with adults, beginning when he was four years old when his mother's colleague assaulted him. A female babysitter touched him when he was nine, and his father's boss sexually abused him for two years from age 12 to 14. His parents had chosen this man to be his surrogate grandfather. Colin also had sexual experiences with his middle brother, Adam, that he found hard to define as abusive. These particular incidents seemed to have a different meaning for him than his sexual contact with others.

Colin felt little emotional connection with his parents, who had separated when he was 16. Colin said nothing about his parents being neglectful. However, his partner, who also attended the interview, described how he could walk through the house bleeding without anyone noticing, suggesting an unusual lack of parental involvement with their children.

Colin had been diagnosed with symptoms of post-traumatic stress disorder (PTSD). He was having difficulties sleeping, and experiencing flashbacks and intrusive thoughts. He believed that society looked down on him as a victim for three main reasons: he was unemployed; he had been sexually abused; and he was suffering from PTSD. He believed that there was a link between being sexually abused, his mental health difficulties and being unemployed.

> From about four to six, a work associate of my mother's, he assaulted me. I have later on found out that he also had a go at both my brothers. My relationship with my next brother down, it's not a good relationship. It's been on and off, on and off. And the reason is that he also abused me. Although I'm not a hundred per cent convinced that he was an abuser as such, 'cause now having that ability to look back and see what was happening with him, I can understand his behaviour to some degree. Recently, I found out things that he'd actually told my grandparents. They decided to do nothing about it. If my grandparents had've done something, perhaps it wouldn't have happened to me, so I bear a bit of resentment towards them.
>
> I've had a fairly chequered past. I was hitchhiking once and I got picked up by an older man in a white Toyota ute. I don't remember a great deal about it. He went out on one of the back roads and paid me for oral sex. I don't have too many issues involving that one. Compared to other stuff that happened it was fairly minor.

I felt a bit shocked when Colin described this incident so calmly, as if it was nowhere near as serious in his own mind as other things that had happened to him in childhood and adolescence. He also described his parents' divorce in very matter-of-fact terms, which made me ponder what we now consider to be 'normal' aspects of family life.

> And then the longest period of abuse I had started when I was 12. And that carried on for two years, when he died, a bloke who was my father's boss. He was sort of given to me as a surrogate grandparent. It turned out that was a bit of a poor judgement on their behalf. I don't know exactly what Mum and Dad know of what happened. I've never spoken to either them about it and Mum's now dead.
>
> And I don't want to speak to my father about it because I bear a lot of resentment to him. Him and I had a fight when I was about 16, and that pretty much set the tone of our relationship. Mum and Dad got divorced and I had to put up with their crap while they were divorcing. I don't really bear much resentment towards them; it was a pretty straightforward divorce. Dad was having an affair and Mum found out. The screaming and yelling was fairly normal, I thought, for what was going on.

Perhaps as a way of taking control of the situation, Colin decided to apply for victim's compensation through the courts. He was finding it difficult to work out who exactly to take to court and he hadn't yet accepted the inevitability of needing to disclose what had actually happened to him publicly and to his family, in order to follow this course of action.

> The only person that I may actually have any chance of taking to court and holding accountable is Mum's work associate. He's the only one that I think the police are actually going to look at. I know that Dad's boss is dead, so they can't really charge anybody. I'm not going to tell the police about my brother because I sort of understand why he did what he did, but it seems I can't forgive what he did.
>
> I don't think I ever consciously forgot [events] or buried them, and never actually thought of them as such. It's just that I dismissed them, ignored them, got busy around them, I just didn't pay any attention to them. When I think back on it, I don't think I ever actually forgot what happened.

Again, Colin's picture of family life struck me forcibly as far from normal. Like many others in this book, he took refuge in drug use from a young age.

> My bedroom wall was full of holes from even before a teenager, I'd punch the wall. In my mid teens I got very carried away with bad choices. I wrote myself off very frequently on pretty much anything I could get my hands on. Didn't use a lot of hallucinogen drugs apart from pot. I smoked a lot of pot. I did try some of the other drugs, tried a bit of speed, a bit of crack, a bit of coke, but I pretty much liked pot, it did the trick for me.

> But then about eight years ago, I had a few life-changing events, which I think is what triggered all the memory back. Mum died and I left my wife and moved in with my partner. I had memories and flashbacks, and I was getting dreams and sounds and sights and crap like that. I spend quite a lot of sleepless nights. I get the night sweats. I'll drench the bed completely. And I've had relationship issues ever since I've had relationships.

Colin showed considerable insight into his own childhood development. He knew that he had been badly affected by events in his childhood and wanted society to pay in some way.

> I'm sick of having to play charades. That period in your teens when you're supposed to build that self-identity, I don't think I've still actually done that as such. The whole arrested development thing, emotionally I'm about a four year old. That was one of the things that prompted me to actually go and get counselling. I wanted to get some control.
>
> The people who did this to me, they were all highly respectable people and got to live their life of luxury, and they've left me in the state where I don't have the tools to go out and achieve what they achieved. I've been unemployed on and off since I left school. Society looks down its nose at me and they're the people that put me here. I feel society let me down. Not any one particular part of it, lots of it did. My parents, the offenders, the Department of Education failed me miserably. I was abused all my school life, and nobody picked up on it. These people are supposed to be trained, paid and trained to do that. So many bits of society failed me that I feel society does owe me to a large degree. It is something that's really starting to piss me off actually, is the fact that people profit off this thing that happened to me, and there ain't no profit in this. This destroys people's lives.

Reluctance by men like Colin to admit to homosexual experiences

Men are often reluctant to admit to having been sexually abused by other men, since there can be a sense of stigma or shame attached to such events, and a fear of being labelled as a homosexual or deviant. Colin was one such man. He had been badly affected by his childhood experiences and he still seemed very angry with everyone involved. He was battling between his desire to tell the police in order to get compensation and his reluctance to disclose the homosexual nature of his experiences. The homosexual nature of his experiences may have added to his anger, given his concern about being stigmatised and labelled as homosexual. His experiences with his brother were somehow different from the others and, while he said that he could understand his brother's behaviour, he couldn't forgive it. He didn't want to expose his brother and yet he wanted to be compensated through the courts. He realised that this would mean telling his family and his children what had happened to him, which was a conundrum.

NARRATIVE OF THE NEED TO REMEMBER AND THE NEED TO FORGET

The common theme between these five stories was the struggle between the desire to forget about childhood memories and the need to remember in order to make sense of life. Hence I have called these stories a *narrative of the need to remember and the need to forget*. I see this narrative as similar to the victim narrative that is so common in the literature, because these men and women were locked in a struggle with the past and unable to move forward in their lives. To a greater or a lesser extent they saw themselves as victims. Hope and Colin saw this as a process of systemic, rather than personal, victimisation. They believed that they had been let down by society, as well as by individual adults. Sylvia, Leo and Tess were living through a period of great distress and rethinking their pasts and their futures, as they grappled with memories of child sexual abuse.

Sylvia and Leo believed that they had experienced such shocking events as children that they had repressed their memories of these events. The need to forget was paramount to their survival. Through therapy, they had realised that they had used out-of-body experiences throughout their adult lives. During the interview they both lost track of what they were saying and, after a few seconds of silence, asked to be reminded about where they were in their story. They both used the word 'dissociation' to describe these experiences. It seemed likely that their narratives had been influenced to some extent by their ongoing life experiences, including therapy. By contrast Tess, Hope and Colin had always remembered what had happened to them but had chosen not to think about it by pushing away or repressing such thoughts.

All five men and women had experienced a need to forget about the past as children and young people. This ability to repress or forget stood them in good stead until, as adults, they were no longer able to maintain the status quo and the need to remember began to surface. Memories and flashbacks started to appear unbidden for Sylvia, Leo and Colin. By contrast, Tess and Hope had always remembered what had happened, but they started to place more importance on their childhood experiences. Remembering became as important as forgetting had been earlier in their lives, because it helped to make sense of many of their life choices. For example, Tess had suppressed all thoughts of her sexual relationship with her stepfather, condoned by her mother, and had only recently put a name to her experiences. This realisation helped her to make sense of many events in her subsequent life.

There was reluctance, even as adults, for these men and women to disclose what had happened to them as children. For Sylvia, Leo and Tess their realisations were too recent. Colin expressed reluctance to talk about his experiences to the police, for fear of negative consequences, whereas Hope didn't believe that she would ever receive justice for the crimes committed against her family. This reluctance to talk about their experiences, except in the privacy of therapy, may be the result of the high level of shame and self-blame experienced by these men and women. It may require an internal shift of some kind before they are able to move beyond these experiences.

These men and women had come to attribute many of the problems they have experienced in their adult lives to their childhood sexual experiences, including feeling suicidal, using drugs and alcohol to excess, and having non-committed sex or sexual encounters with men and women outside the context of a stable relationship. Hope said very little about what she believed had been the impact of her own rape by a neighbour. She tended to speak much more generally about the impact of paedophiles on children, rather than refer to her own experiences.

Sylvia, Tess and Leo had what could be described as a fragile sense of their own identity. Sylvia was discovering that she had a gaping hole inside herself, which she had covered up with a mask of normality. Tess carried so much confusion about her mother's behaviour that she was left doubting herself as a mother. Leo believed that he had fragmented into many different parts when he was very young. He oscillated between wanting to reintegrate these parts of himself and deciding that it was safest to remain childlike.

Hope and Colin described how they continued to suffer as a result of their childhood experiences. They both saw child sexual abuse as endemic in our society and were determined to eradicate it. They had gradually become campaigners for the rights of others. In this way they had salvaged a more positive sense of self from their own experiences.

A transitional narrative?

There is a sense in which Hope and Colin could have been seen as telling a *narrative of justice at any cost*, in that they were developing through their pursuit of social justice and perhaps finding some existential meaning to their suffering. However, they were still very much embroiled in their childhood experiences and unable to move on. Unlike the women described in the following two chapters, they had not become professional helpers of others or completed the process of seeking justice or breaking the cycle of abuse.

However, the *narrative of the need to remember and the need to forget* may be transitional in nature. We know that many people move from a period of ongoing suffering to a more optimistic period in their lives. For example, Jewels, who you will meet in the next chapter, recovered memories of child sexual abuse but was able to move from seeing herself as a victim to seeing how she had grown and been transformed through the recovery process. There are many examples in the literature of people moving from thinking of themselves as victims to seeing themselves as survivors of child sexual abuse. Given this process of transition from one narrative to another, it is possible to be optimistic that some people currently telling a *narrative of the need to remember and the need to forget* might eventually be able to look back and see that they had gained strength from their adversity and been transformed as a result.

In the next chapter we meet three women who overcame incestuous experiences in childhood to become protectors and helpers of others.

SUMMARY

Key points
- The narratives told by these five men and women were of the profound ongoing suffering that they experienced as a result of their childhood sexual experiences. Their narratives were similar to many of the victim narratives found in the literature.
- Some had forgotten or repressed their childhood experiences, only to remember them as adults. Others had always remembered, wanted to remember and campaigned against child abuse. Hence their narratives have been described as *the need to remember and the need to forget.*
- Piecing together what had happened to them as children helped to explain some of the chaos and the choices that they had made in their adult lives.
- Their experiences had left Sylvia, Tess and Leo feeling vulnerable and fragmented, without a strong sense of identity.
- Hope and Colin demonstrated a level of resilience by becoming campaigners for others in the fight against systemic victimisation and child sexual abuse.
- There was a sense in which these men and women were still embroiled in a struggle with their pasts and were unable to move forward in their lives.
- It is possible that this is a transitional narrative and that most people are eventually able to tell a more optimistic and transformational narrative about their childhood experiences.

CHAPTER 6

Protecting and helping others

INTRODUCTION

Chapter aims
- Tell the narratives of three women who felt proud of the fact that they worked to protect others and to help survivors of child sexual abuse.
- Describe the ways in which they believed that their incestuous childhood sexual experiences had affected them.
- Examine their coping mechanisms including dissociation.
- Outline how they developed a strong sense of themselves as protectors and helpers of others.

This chapter explores the ways in which three women faced their childhood adversity and were transformed in the process. They all chose to protect other people within their family. These women all went on to work in the helping professions. Even though they would have preferred not to have had the experiences that they did, they felt transformed by them to a certain extent.

These women's experiences in childhood included both physical and emotional abuse within their families. For Jewels and Heather, their sexual contact with adults started when they were very young and lasted for an average of four years, whereas Emm's experience of sexual abuse was a single incident with her father. These women were aware of the major impacts that these experiences had on their lives and could have been included in the previous chapter. However, they seemed to have come to terms more with their childhood experiences. They didn't feel that their experiences explained everything that had happened to them or had ruined their lives, but rather that they had been able to adapt and learn from them. They would have preferred not to have had to go through this process, but believed that they had emerged stronger as a result.

PROTECTING MYSELF AND OTHERS IN THE FAMILY

Jewels, Emm and Heather had overcome their incestuous childhood experiences and other forms of child maltreatment, mainly by developing a sense of themselves as protecting other family members. They developed a strong identity for themselves over the years, overcoming their challenging upbringings. Jewels and Heather had out-of-body experiences in childhood, and had been fearful and angry as adolescents. All three women didn't tell anyone about what happened to them. For Heather in particular, this decision was the beginning of her empowerment as a protector of others.

Some people moved from one narrative to another during the course of their lives. For example, when she was an adult Jewels had remembered being sexually abused by her father and by other men. If interviewed earlier in her life she would probably have described her ongoing suffering and been included in the previous chapter. However, she appeared to have transcended her childhood maltreatment and had come to see herself as called to be a healer of others. This is a theme that runs throughout the stories of these three women.

Jewels' story – 'cut off at the throat'

Jewels was a slim, somewhat nervous woman, with clear blue eyes. She was elegantly dressed and wrapped in a beautiful, colourful shawl. She was an unemployed woman in her late forties, living in a rural community. She had one son who mostly lived with his father. Throughout her adult life she struggled with drug and relationship problems. About four years previously, in therapy, she had recovered memories of being sexually abused. This involved sexual contact with a stranger, her grandfather and a neighbour, all between the ages of three and seven. When her father found out about the neighbour, he initially threatened her but later had sexual intercourse with her, too.

Jewels also remembered sexual experiences with her older brother, her cousins, and boys at school. She got involved in drugs aged 19, moving quickly from an addiction to marijuana and alcohol to a heroin addiction. She had relationships with a series of dominating men. She described having suicidal thoughts, up to a few months before the interview. Jewels was angry with both her parents and felt particularly betrayed by her mother. However, she didn't want to confront them.

Most of the people that I interviewed started telling their stories beginning in childhood, whereas Jewels started her story in the middle and then went backwards, as she described the things that she had remembered about her childhood as an adult. In a way this was a story about remembering, rather than revisiting childhood experiences. There were times when Jewels herself seemed unsure whether or not she believed her own memories.

I can remember my brother trying to have sex with me when I was about

13 or 14. He was a couple of years older. I yelled and he just called me a bitch and left. And there were just early experiences with my cousins. And I can remember at school at the age of 12, being molested by boys and not feeling I had any way of defending myself, just having to sit there and accept it.

Jewels told a sad story of multiple abuses. She exemplified many women who are incest victims. They often see themselves as different from other women, 'not normal', and are afraid that they will be bad mothers to their own children. They develop a very negative self-image and can become self-destructive, leaving themselves open to re-victimisation. For example, some have unwanted pregnancies, enter relationships with violent or emotionally abusive men, submit to being raped or physically abused, become addicted to drugs or alcohol, or attempt suicide.[1] This applies to both men and women.[2] Victims of incest committed by a father or brother seem to be particularly affected, possibly as a result of being objectified sexually. Certainly, Jewels had several of these experiences.

And when I was about 19 I got involved in drugs, first marijuana, alcohol and then into the hard drugs, heroin. I had a lot of sexual experiences at the time, and I wasn't able to say no. I just neatly fell into the passive–submissive role. I used to pick dominating men and expect them to be my protector and make all the decisions, and often I would end up being abused. I was in one relationship where he did force sex on me a number of times, including anally, and where he did also hit me once. But that wasn't really a common experience. Normally, I'd just submit anyway.

I felt sad as Jewels described how she would submit to men sexually. However, I recognised this behaviour, since many female incest survivors develop negative ideas about their gender identity or their sexual selves, either withdrawing from sexual activity or engaging in it in a compulsive way.[3] Some describe themselves as 'unworthy, never good enough', with an 'excessive need to please', with 'something wrong with me', 'to blame for all my problems', with 'problems in relationships' and 'different from others'.[4]

I realised that there was a lot of anger in me and I just, and I was terrified of that anger. It was just like I was going to explode. If I let it out there's just going to be a massive explosion. And so I used the drugs in many ways to keep the anger down, to keep what I felt was a lot of pain down. My health started to really suffer and I was diagnosed with hepatitis C.

About four years ago the memories started to surface. A lot of them were disjointed. I started to see images. Something happened when I was about three, which appeared to be a rape by a teenage boy, which was very quick. There were memories that my grandfather started to have sex with me when I was about five. My mother was very overburdened with three children, the last one retarded, and she was only 22. The affection that I got from my grandfather, even though it was sex, fulfilled that need for touch for me.

At the time of the interview I believed Jewels' story even though it had a melo-dramatic quality to it. But as I listened to the tape recording and thought about it all, I started to doubt that it was literally true. However, I still believe that it represents a psychological truth about her family.[5]

And then there was this memory of this man living under the house, a foreign man. I came to realise that it was actually my father. He was a butcher. He threatened me with a butcher's knife, threatening to cut out my vagina because of what he'd found me doing [having sex with the neighbour]. And then he lost control and started having sex with me. It seemed to end when I was about seven. And then the memories were just lost, totally lost.

I felt guilty about my inability to accept the veracity of Jewels' story. Her story sounded similar to other stories that I had heard in therapy, told by clients who were in extreme pain, having recovered memories of childhood incest. I wanted to believe Jewels, but a part of me found this impossible. However, I could empathise with her pain and her difficulties in the world. Despite a lot of hard work in therapy, Jewels still felt dirty, ashamed and responsible for what had happened to her. She wanted to connect more with her body and her emotions, but dissociation and drug use had become protective habits for her.

There's a belief that I don't have a right to say no to men, that I have to submit, their needs are more important than mine. I've realised in the last few years that I just don't seem to inhabit my body. It's like I've been cut off at the throat and just been very out of touch with my feelings and my pain, with my anger, just really lived in my head. And the marijuana, that more or less was a tool to keep me there. Whenever I tried to get off the drugs, after a while a feeling would start to surface, and I'd straight away go back to smoke to push it all down.

I thought it was interesting that Jewels used the metaphor of being 'cut off at the throat' to describe the disconnection between her mind and her body, her thoughts and her feelings. This metaphor echoed her recovered memory of being threatened with a knife by her father, the butcher. She also described a metaphorical meeting between herself as an adult and herself as a child, when the memories from her childhood started to surface.

After years of just having to silence it, because everything that happened was my fault, I was responsible for it, I was dirty, I was evil. And so I had to keep it quiet. And when it surfaced, I really wanted to be heard. And when the memories first started to come up, I went looking for me as a small child. I found her hiding in a dungeon. And I know this is only metaphorical but that's where I found her, hiding down in this dungeon, underground down these stairs, with rats and dirt and darkness, and she was just so dirty and so untidy, and so full of anger and pain and terror.

When she started to remember her past, Jewels often felt overwhelmed with anger towards her parents. She felt violated and betrayed by her father and unprotected by her mother and, hardly surprisingly, found it hard to trust people. She also found it hard to trust herself and experienced an ongoing battle with mental illness.

> There's always been a lot of rage and anger at my parents. I've never really been able to relate to them; I've never had a great deal of respect for them. I've never had trust of men or trust of woman. I feel that there's this sense that my mother abandoned me, that she allowed it to happen. She betrayed me and I felt as though I was betrayed by men, too, and used by them. And there's just still the doubt with it. Is this just all in my imagination? Did this really happen?
>
> I have this total fear of orgasm, this inability to let go. For years I just couldn't get anywhere near it, and now I approach it and then there's just this terror. I just go into my head and back off totally. When I was a little child, I was stimulated and there's this terror of having orgasm or showing that I did enjoy it, and that still seems to be with me. And I've always had this sense that I didn't want to be here, that I just want to be off this planet. I just want to be dead, and I've had bouts of quite severe depression and suicide thoughts.

Jewels recognised that she had played the role of a victim for too long and had started to see herself more like a survivor than a victim. This was helped by her vision of herself as able to heal others.

> I've always had a victim attitude all my life. But I don't have to be victimised, I don't have to see myself as powerless. I am a strong capable woman, and it is safe for me to be a woman. So I have a dream, a goal of being able to eventually, as I heal myself, being able to start reaching out to other people, and helping other people through this journey. So I think I've been given a purpose in life that I never had before. So it's almost like the alchemist transforming the lead into gold.

Jewels no longer a victim but a healer

In the past Jewels felt a great deal of shame about what had happened to her and clung to the role of victim. Dissociation, coupled with use of drugs and alcohol, was a powerful combination that protected Jewels from feeling any anger or pain. Coming off drugs led to a resurfacing of her feelings, which in turn led to using drugs to push the feelings back down. Jewels described this cycle that she had been through several times and how drug use enabled men to victimise her further.

More recently, Jewels had become determined to stop thinking of herself as a victim and to become the strong, capable woman that she knew she could be. She had learned to say no as an adult, to interrupt the vicious cycle of choosing to enter abusive relationships with men. Like many other people who had abusive childhoods, Jewels felt a calling to work as a healer. She loved living and working in the Australian bush, surrounded by nature. She was on a powerful healing journey and was going through a transformation. Her long-term goal was to help other people to achieve this transformation for themselves. In this way, she was similar to Emm who had become a child advocate.

Emm's story – 'at least I had someone'

Emm was a soft-spoken woman in her late thirties, married with children. She told the story of her childhood experiences with a cruel, violent and neglectful mother and an alcoholic father. In a family of four children, Emm and her older brother were tied to the clothes-line by her mother and left outside to play in cold weather. She described being hit by her mother on several occasions, and trying to hide in a cupboard.

Emm always felt close to her father whereas her brother was close to her mother. As an adult Emm believed she needed her relationship with her father to ensure her survival. One night when she was about eight her father came home drunk and kissed her in a sexualised way. She found this experience terrifying and lay in bed, stiff as a board, hoping that he would leave her alone. Emm felt guilty for pretending to be asleep, which she knew was wrong. She found the whole incident totally confusing and, in that sense, consistent with all her other childhood experiences. As an adult, she puzzled over whether it was worse than the other forms of childhood maltreatment she received. She had recently discovered that one of her twin sisters had also had a similar sexual experience with their father. This had changed its meaning and made her question whether she had, in fact, had a special bond with him after all.

> My older brother was Mum's, and I am equally Dad's. It's unspoken but indisputable fact of the family. And the poor twins, they were nobody's. They were really [sighs] unwanted and named as such. My mother used to tie my brother and I to the clothes-line, so that we didn't escape. I think her primary motivation

was safety, but she didn't want us inside. And this city was very cold so I have some really vivid memories of being very cold. But I also have some really happy memories, tied to the clothes-line.

One day I put a jar down heavily and she turned on me. She hit and kicked the living shit out of me, and I was really badly bruised. What always amazes me when she did this, there were never bruises where people could see. So there was a measure of cruelty about Mum that was quite deliberate. She didn't usually hit me when Dad was around. Another time I was bleeding from the back of my head, because she'd cut me with her wedding ring and the back of my legs were burnt because I'd been pushed against the oil heater. It's no fucking wonder I work in child protection.

Emm told me the story of her mother's cruelty in a calm, almost serene, manner. I found it distressing to imagine her and her brother tied to a clothes-line, fearful of being beaten or kicked by their mother. Emm seemed to be far more disturbed by her mother's cruelty and violence than by her father's sexualised behaviour towards her under the influence of alcohol. In fact she was close to her father, and dependent on him for protection against her mother.

He is so bad and yet he was really all there was. And she was cruel; she still is cruel. I wish she wasn't cruel; if she was just bad or unreliable, it would have been a lot easier. The bulk of the violence, it actually went from Mum to Dad. Dad was burnt through to the bone on the arm by an iron. I wasn't there for that incident, thank goodness. Mum said to me it was self-defence. Apparently, Dad returned home drunk, and she'd locked the door, and he took an axe and busted the door down. And she defended herself with the iron.

Mum was very unpredictable, very unavailable, and Dad was nice to be around. And the only memory I have of Dad being sexual towards me is so minor, but it is the relationship and the context of growing up with no choice really but to be close to Dad. And I liked being close to Dad, that's the most painful thing about it.

One night Dad was kneeled down next to the bed. I might have been seven or eight. This drunken stuff about 'Your poor old father' and 'Haven't you got a kiss for your poor old father?' And when he kissed me it was not like a peck on the cheek, and I had never been kissed like that before. It was really scary, he kissed me on the lips and his mouth was open, and it was a long time, it wasn't a goodnight kiss. And I just wanted him to go away. But he wouldn't, he just carried on with this drunken drivel and about how I didn't love him and I just kept trying to pretend I was asleep. I felt really as if I was lying, and I knew lying was bad. So I felt absolutely torn, I knew I was doing the wrong thing by pretending I was asleep.

Rather than dissociation, Emm described a changing process of initially recalling her experience with her father and automatically pushing the thoughts into her subconscious. Over time she was able to suppress the thoughts deliberately until she was ready to deal with them. Growing up in her particular family had been extremely confusing. It was only when she was in a good enough position in her life that she felt able to examine that confusion.

> I've always known it, but it's only in more recent years able to be looked at. Even say three years ago, I would say, 'Okay, I know you're there,' and shove it away. It was a more conscious shoving away, and before that it was more automatically shoved away. Back then, everything was shoved away, like nothing made sense. I can honestly say that, coming out of adolescence and into my early twenties, I could probably register one emotion and it was confusion.

I was surprised to hear of Emm's dramatic somatic reaction as an adolescent, when her father was rushed into hospital requiring emergency surgery. She retired to bed with a severe pain and was physically unable to move until her father returned home. She explained this as her body demonstrating what she knew emotionally, that her survival depended on her father and that she could not function without him. It demonstrated the power of the mind to affect the body and the strength of her need for her father.

> [When Dad was hospitalised] I went to bed with a pain in my side and couldn't, not didn't, couldn't get up. I was there sick for about a week, until we heard that he was going to be alright. But that still floors me. I only understand how important it was for me to have Dad, through knowing that my body did that. And I can honestly tell you I couldn't get up, and they told me there was nothing wrong physically. But I was literally struck down. So the relationship with Dad was terribly important. If my life depended on Mum, I'd be dead. It's just that simple.

Emm struggled to understand her childhood experiences, even as an adult. She recognised that she had chosen to believe what she needed to believe as a child, in order to survive.

> I can't deny that I was terrified that night, absolutely stiff. Is it worse than the drinking? Is it worse than the violence? Is it worse than his emotional stuff? In some ways it's more repungant [sic] and repulsive, and personally violating. It is, but it still gets pushed into the realms of 'at least I had someone'. It feels devastating as an adult, but it actually would have been devastating as a child to put this together; it would have killed me. In some ways the truth is the truth. He'll die, she'll die. But when I was a child, there was a sense of only letting those things be true that would get you through.

Emm's choice to believe what was helpful

Emm didn't say this, but I sensed that what had really frightened her about her father's behaviour was what might have developed, rather than what had actually happened. She knew as a child that she was reliant on him for her survival. Emm described a form of childlike, magical thinking that protected her from knowing the truth about him. She knew that she needed her father's care to keep her alive so, as a child, she chose to believe in him. She could now see that it would have been too devastating for her to realise that, in reality, she couldn't depend on either parent. What made this all so complex for Emm was that she knew that if he had gone further sexually with her, she would still have needed him. But all this paled into insignificance compared to her mother's physical cruelty towards her. The level of violence between her parents was similar to that between Heather's parents.

Heather's story – 'the core that's you'

Heather was a lively, quick-witted woman in her early forties, living in a small rural town, with her three children and her female partner. Her father was a violent alcoholic, who hit his wife and children. Heather described her unstable family background and the domestic violence that she witnessed as a small child, which had a profound impact on her. She was sexually abused by her father until the age of nine, when her parents separated. Heather took on the role of protector within the family, in the hope of sparing her siblings from sexual abuse.

Heather always sided with her mother, against her violent father. As an adult, Heather's husband told her mother that she was a lesbian and about the sexual abuse. Heather's mother refused to believe her and accused her of making false accusations against her father, because of her sexuality. They had since broken off contact and Heather was still trying to understand this complex relationship.

> I'm one of six children, three boys and then three girls. We grew up with a father who was abusive, violent, always in debt, gambling, inflicted horrific injuries on my mother. And we stayed there till I was about nine. We were always having to hide cut-throat razor blades, and bullets and things like that, and being shoved out windows as a small child to ring the police.
>
> I was his favourite. You always push forward to get favours for the others. You knew what was going to happen, but you'd protect your sisters, because if he wasn't doing it with me, he was going to do it with them. If I could smooth him over, or divert him then the violence would dissipate. Or if he was getting drunk, and my other sisters were in the room, we had bunks in one bedroom, and I always slept on the bottom bunk, just to protect them, because I thought, 'Well, if he's not going to get it from me, where else is he going to get it? He'll start on my younger sister.'

This was a familiar story, that of protecting siblings from the same fate. It was very important to Heather that she was able to protect her siblings from being sexually abused. She also tried to protect her mother from being beaten by her father when she was little, and was very relieved when they separated. She and her siblings were terrified of his violent outbursts. Heather found his violent behaviour hard to understand and believed that it impacted on her more than the sexual abuse.

> Nothing's ever talked about in my family, everything's always under the mat. Even the domestic violence. It was just bizarre. My mother actually decided to leave that relationship. She'd be dead if she didn't; I have no doubt about that. My brothers used to sleep with steel bars under their pillows. We used to move around a lot, so I went to something like nine schools. So my mother decided to leave. I think she knew about the whole situation, I've no doubt about that.

Like other incest victims, Heather avoided intimate relationships. I was struck by the way that she saw relationships as either abusive or non-abusive – this had become her way of viewing the world.

> You just don't cope with it as a kid. You get out of that environment, you're so grateful to be out of it. So you do learn to disassociate [sic] which helps you cope. It is just a coping mechanism and it may not be a good one, but it gets you through. In my teenage years I sort of avoided relationships, particularly intimate relationships. I threw myself into sport in a big way. I just thought that sex didn't interest me, having grown up in this heterosexual world, and never been exposed to any other forms of sexuality. There was heterosexual sex, which could be abusive or not abusive. That was my framework probably.

Like many other incest victims, Heather became sexually active at a young age. When her first child was born with a disability, she looked deep within herself to work out who she really was and what she really stood for. She was forced to deal with her new role as a mother, as well as her own feelings of grief about her own upbringing.

> I got involved with one of my teachers when I was 15. He was early thirties. It was all hidden, it was cloak and dagger stuff. I ended up marrying this guy. It was like just a going through the motions. There was never a big focus on sex so that suited me. We'd be in bed having sex and I'd be miles away. It was just like a sex worker. My first child had a disability so I was thrust into the world of healthcare unfortunately. And that was a very difficult time, because a lot of stuff came up, just trying to deal with your own baggage. So I really had to dig deep within myself to work out who I was, for the first time in my life.

Heather realised that her life had been profoundly affected by her childhood. She had suffered from depression for many years, had suicidal thoughts from time to time, and used alcohol as an escape. She hated the idea of being a blood relative to her father.

> Suicide the whole thing, been there, done that. Particularly as a teenager, thinking that that bastard's blood ran through my veins in terms of abuse, and God, I used to drink myself to death practically. I was paralytic, bloody 95 per cent of the time. Thank God syringes weren't around because I would have done it.

Heather didn't believe that her childhood sexual experiences had any impact on her sexuality. She didn't believe that women became lesbians after being sexually abused by men. However, coming out had been a painful experience because it had coincided with her ex-husband revealing to her mother that she had been sexually abused by her father. Her mother chose not to believe Heather, denied that incest had ever taken place, and accused Heather of fabricating the whole story. She declared her to be mentally ill and tried to prevent her from gaining custody of her own children. Heather experienced this as a devastating betrayal by the woman she had tried so hard to protect as a child.

> It wasn't really until I went to university [again] that I even had my eyes open to what gay was. I didn't even know it existed. By the time I finished my degree, I had no doubt that I was a lesbian. When the family found out I was involved with a woman, it was just the whole shebang. I ended up saying to my husband about my father's abuse. And so he goes off and tells my mother. So it was, 'I must have been imagining it' and 'That's why I was gay' because you know I was sick or I had a mental health problem, or I was just queer or weird.
>
> I was so loyal to my mother and the one time that I needed her, she told me she'd prefer it if I was dead. I couldn't understand that betrayal. It's very complex, or intricate unravelling of this dynamic between this child who was the mother's protector, and the mother actually manipulating the child. It's manipulation by rejection; it's like a sick type of engagement.

Heather disliked the fact that, in her opinion, there was a strong societal belief that victims of child sexual abuse were damaged, inferior and tainted. She rejected this and chose to see herself instead as a worthwhile human being, who had tried to protect her siblings and her mother from harm. As it became more socially acceptable to discuss childhood maltreatment in public, it became even harder for Heather to feel that her individual experiences would be honoured and understood. Heather felt angry that some victims exploited their situation, thereby trivialising and minimising the experiences of others.

> I feel that it's been minimalised in a sense. If you say you were sexually abused as a child, 'Oh, well, so was everyone else.' Like we've got to the point in our society where we don't really think that it's all that traumatic any more. I think people come out and say they were or they weren't for attention, so it trivialises what we've been through.
>
> There's certainly a lot of conjecture out there that all lesbians are abused as children, blah, blah, blah. A lot of them were because they're women [laughs]. Hello! But there certainly is that connotation out there from a broader community perspective that if you were abused as child then, chances are that you're going to hate men or you're not going to want to have anything to do with them. You're seen as dirty. She's a lesser being because she's been tarnished. So people look down their noses at her. You were abused as a child therefore you're no good.

I admired Heather and the way that she had found the courage to come forward to be interviewed, even though this was obviously a painful process for her. She had realised that she had a core being that no one could touch or destroy. She had turned her own life around without help or support from her family, by relying on her inner strength born of adversity. Her role as a protector of her sisters and her mother was very important to her self-concept.

> But the only thing that people can't attack is what's inside. It's like you are having this steel rod that's surrounded by things that no one can touch. There's always something in you that is your own, and you're your own person, despite what anyone does to you, you still have this core that's you. And nothing that anyone can do can change that.

Heather's rejection of dominant cultural narrative as 'damaged goods'

Women who have experienced incest cannot explain their experiences to themselves or to others in terms of the traditional, cultural stories of kind fathers and their beloved daughters. As a result, they often tend to blame themselves for what has happened. Feelings of low self-esteem and self-blame can lead girls to make poor choices in their intimate lives, which may leave them vulnerable to further re-victimisation. It can be difficult to separate out how much of the trauma associated with child sexual abuse and rape is caused by sexual violence and how much is caused by societal and cultural beliefs, such as the belief that if a woman is raped she becomes damaged goods.[6]

Heather hated this kind of thinking. She rejected the idea that she was damaged goods and felt angry with other 'victims' for talking publicly about their experiences and diminishing her as a result. Heather felt silenced by these societal attitudes. I felt honoured that she had come forward to be interviewed, despite her fear that I might somehow see her as tarnished or dirty as a consequence of her childhood experiences.

NARRATIVE OF PROTECTING AND HELPING OTHERS

This chapter describes how three women faced their childhood adversity. They were all able to see that they had been transformed by their experiences and had emerged as stronger women as a result. They felt good about the way they had overcome the hardships of the past. In particular, they felt good about the way they had been able to protect other children from harm. Apart from Heather, whose story was told to her family by her ex-husband, the other two women had chosen not to confront their victimisers or to tell family members about their experiences.

Jewels and Heather described a number of difficulties in their adult lives which they attributed to their childhood sexual experiences within the family. Emm had experienced problems only in adolescence. Although these women described many difficulties that they had faced, they were all at a point in their lives where they were functioning well and felt that they had overcome most of these problems, including excessive drug and alcohol use, and physical and sexual problems. The lingering problem seemed to be depression and suicidal thoughts that both Jewels and Heather continued to experience in adulthood.

These three women had taken on the role of protecting and helping others. Jewels had decided to become a healer of others, whereas Emm and Heather already worked in the helping professions. Heather had tried to protect her mother and her younger siblings from her father's unpredictable, violent and abusive behaviour. And Jewels and Emm had both decided not to confront their parents about what had happened. They had chosen to protect others by remaining silent, rather than by speaking out. Heather's story helps to explain this choice. She believed that speaking out publicly would mean that she would be stigmatised as a victim of child sexual abuse and seen as a lesser person as a result. She chose to be protective of herself and her family instead.

In the next chapter, three more women describe how they were also transformed by their childhood experiences. They made different choices with regard to speaking out in adulthood. They decided to seek justice despite the enormous personal cost to themselves, in terms of loss of connection with their families. They made this difficult decision in the hope of protecting children from abuse in the future.

SUMMARY

Key points

- The narratives told by these three women spoke of the suffering that they experienced as a result of their incestuous childhood experiences.
- However, they chose to tell a *narrative of protecting and helping others,*

having found a positive sense of who they were. As children, they suffered in silence to protect other family members. As adults, they preferred to remain silent and had all chosen to work in the helping professions.

- They demonstrated great resilience in overcoming their incestuous childhood experiences.
- These women described how they had been transformed by their childhood adversity into better, stronger women who had been able to protect others from harm.

CHAPTER 7

Justice at any cost

INTRODUCTION

Chapter aims

- Tell the narratives of three women who felt proud of the fact that, as adults, they had brought their victimisers to justice in order to protect other children.
- Describe the ways in which they believed that their incestuous experiences in childhood had affected them.
- Explore how they tried to tell of their abuse as children and how this may have influenced their desire to seek justice as adults.
- Outline how they developed a strong sense of themselves as seeking justice, at considerable personal cost.

This chapter explores the ways in which three women faced their incestuous childhood experiences by reporting their victimisers to the police, in an attempt to make meaning out of suffering and to protect future generations. Even though they would have preferred not to have had the experiences that they did, they had been transformed by them. These women's experiences included sexual abuse throughout their childhood and both physical and emotional abuse.

SEEKING JUSTICE AND BREAKING THE CYCLE

Karen, Tina and Jane were sexually assaulted by members of their family for as long as eight years. Karen and Jane both had fathers who were physically, emotionally and sexually abusive. They had all reported their victimisers to the police as adults, and were willing to accept the consequences of this action. In all three cases their families sided with the victimiser and, eventually, these women were forced to cut off contact with family members. This was a double blow for them. However, they did not regret what they had done. In fact they were proud of their actions and felt that they had grown stronger as a result of the ordeal that they had been through. Seeking justice had been their way of facing up to their childhood adversity.

Jane could also be described as a protector of others. She had a strong need to protect her twin sister from experiencing any pain. She definitely identified herself as a protector of her twin, and in that respect her story was similar to those of Jewels, Emm and Heather. However, Jane did not want to help other people in general. Her main passion was to prevent other children from being sexually abused and to open their mothers' eyes as to what was happening in the family. For her, justice and breaking the cycle of abuse had become more important than protecting others, hence her inclusion in this chapter.

Karen's story – 'the lucky one'

Karen was an attractive, slim woman in her early forties, with three children. She was brought up on a farm as one of five children with a violent, alcoholic father. She had difficulty with reading at school and was severely belted if she got a word wrong. The children were isolated from other children and never allowed to have friends home. Karen's father molested her from the ages of four to 13, when she stood up to him and told her mother what he had been doing.

After this, Karen's mother asked her if she wanted her father to leave home. Karen didn't want to upset her mother so she said he could stay. He continued to abuse her physically but not sexually. Karen later found out that he had sexually abused all of his children, including her brother. As a child she knew what had happened to one sister, because her father had sex with them together on one occasion. Both girls knew that the safest thing to do at the time was to bury that knowledge and never to speak of it to anyone.

Karen described herself as promiscuous in adolescence. She became pregnant at 16 and had a termination. In her thirties she and her sisters told the police about their childhood experiences. Her mother supported her father throughout the trial. He went to jail for three years for physically abusing them, and died there. Karen had an amazing ability to remain positive despite her upbringing. She saw herself as the 'lucky one' because she hadn't succumbed to drugs, alcohol or mental illness despite her ordeal.

> Well, my experience started when I was four, and I can remember it just like it was yesterday. It's just like putting a video in the video player and just watching it. I can see the bedroom, everything. My father caressed me, the whole bit. Me thinking, 'Wow, hey, I'm getting attention, this is amazing.' He first told me that 'This is something between you and me. This is secret. Not to tell Mummy.' He asked me if I would touch his penis. And I said, 'No, I'm not allowed to do that.' And he said, 'I'm saying that it's okay.' He actually made me fondle him and he then tried to make me give him oral sex.

> When I was younger 'it was a secret'. As I got older it was 'You tell your mum anything and I'll belt the hell out of you,' or 'I'll kill you.' So I was petrified. There was mental abuse, physical abuse. So that put fear in us. I was petrified. My sister, who is 18 months older, he had us in a session together. And it was completely forgotten afterwards. We said, 'Okay, that's it. We are never, ever to speak about this.' We didn't actually talk about it until I was 20. That's when I found out he'd done it to my other sister and everybody else including my brother. So he went from one to the other, to the other, to the other.

Karen was brought up in a house ruled by fear. Her father used typical abusive tactics[1] and grooming behaviour,[2] beginning by telling his daughter that what they were doing was a secret and going on to threaten her if she told anyone. Not only was her father physically and sexually abusive towards his children but he was also psychologically cruel towards them. His tactics worked when they were young.

> I've got a phobia of Christmas beetles because when I was only little a Christmas beetle flew into the bath and I screamed. He belted me and then put me in a towel out the front. There were swarms of Christmas beetles, under the light, and they were crawling all over me. And he made me stand out the front for a good half hour. You tend to remember more of the beltings than what you remember of the sexual part of it.

One day Karen blurted out the story in front of her mother, but nothing really changed. Her father stopped sexually abusing her but continued to be violent towards her, and punished her for telling. Karen believed that she had done the right thing, but she hated the fact that he continued to sexually abuse her sisters.

> I was getting bad marks at school so I ran away to a friend's place. He come and picked us up, saying, 'You're dead when you get home. You are going to have the biggest belting you've ever had.' And I've had beltings where I've been bruised from ankle to neck, welts, purple welts. He hit me twice and I had enough guts to say, 'If youse [sic] hit me once more, I'm going to tell Mum.'
>
> Mum said, 'Do you want him to stay? Or do you want him to go?' Well, what does a 13-year-old kid want most in their life, is the family to be happy? And I couldn't imagine me saying for him to go, because then my mum would have hated me. So I had all this pressure put on me to say, 'Well, he can stay.' Then he proceeded to belt me, and she let him do it.

I found it interesting that Karen chose to see herself as still a virgin, when she had sex with a boy of her own age at 14. Her father described her as 'the biggest slut in the world' and Karen seemed to have accepted his very negative view of her. Like many other children who have been sexually abused, she internalised feelings of blame for what had happened to her.

> I lost my virginity at 14, but it wasn't special, it wasn't anything. It just was to some bloke at school. I suppose I acted like a true hussy, just done anything, slept with anybody. Then at 16, I fell pregnant and I had that aborted, because I was just too young. So from when I was 18 I didn't have a mother and father any more. But it was the best thing I ever did [leaving home to get married].

Once people knew that she had taken her father to court, Karen also had to contend with gossip. 'She's been abused. She'll probably abuse her kids. And don't leave your kids with her because she'll abuse them as well.' Other mothers saw her as a potential victimiser, although she argued that she was most unlikely to hurt another child, having gone through the experience herself. I admired her outspokenness.

> My way of dealing with this was to talk. I'd tell anybody. Just so that it made me feel better. Nobody would leave their kids with me. I'm positive that they would think that I'd do something to harm their children. But that was the furtherest [sic] thing from my mind. The crap about 'Oh if you've been abused, you're going to be an abuser' that is absolute crap as far as I'm concerned.
>   I told the police and it was like 'Wow, I've done it,' and 'Oh, I'm scared.' I more or less slapped myself, 'You idiot, Karen, you're a grown up. You don't have to worry. He's done wrong. You've done nothing wrong.' It was like everything was just lifted off my shoulders, of this secret that's been held in for so long. I've told somebody that's going to do something about it. Everybody else I told didn't do anything about it.

I was fascinated that, even in this day and age, the sisters were willing to protect their brother from his story coming out into the open. They seemed to accept that it would have been worse for a man than for a woman for others to know that he had been sexually abused as a child by his father, perhaps because of the homosexual nature of the act. Karen didn't agree with his decision, but she respected it at the time.

> My brother didn't want to be involved with the court case. If it had've gone to the media, well for him to feel that he could hold his head up, because he's got a business of his own. Like I don't see the difference between a man and a woman. My way of dealing with this, it's better to be out in the open, encourage other people that this has happened to, to come out and say something, not to hide it. He's hiding it.

> My sisters and I went through court. My mother had the opportunity to
> redeem herself, but she sat with him all the way through the court hearing. And
> she had to hear everything that he'd done to us, all the itty, nitty, gritty bits. He
> died in jail. When I heard I let out this humungous 'Yippee'. And it was like
> 'Wow', like justice. It was what we wanted. I wanted him dead, but he needed to
> stay in jail a bit longer, then die just before he was about to come out.

Karen was very honest about her inability to protect her sisters from harm. She
felt bad about it, but she also recognised that she needed to protect herself too
as a child. I admired the way she had faced her ordeal.

> I didn't protect my little sister. My big sister feels the same way. She says, 'I didn't
> protect my brother and sisters. How am I supposed to live with myself? I knew
> what was going on.' But you just think, 'No, I don't want anybody to hurt me.
> I've had enough hurt. I've got to protect me!' A lot of people have said to me,
> 'How come you're not in the loony bin?' I honestly don't know, couldn't tell
> you. Just the lucky one I suppose.

As an adult, Karen felt good that she had been able to send her father to jail.
Even though it had severed her relationships with her mother, grandmother and
brother, she still felt that it was worthwhile. It was empowering for her to go
to court and win. Karen's siblings found the court case very stressful and most
became clinically depressed afterwards. However, Karen went from strength to
strength. She felt good about the outcome, which bolstered her self-confidence,
and was proud of her capacity for survival.

For Karen, disclosure was as traumatic as the abuse itself

Disclosure of child sexual abuse has been described as a process that can be very
traumatic for the child. Trauma can be experienced by the child before, during
and after the sexual contact, and can be related as much to the act of telling as
to the abuse itself. Much of the stigmatisation happens after the disclosure when
the child experiences the reactions of family members and friends.[3] This was
certainly true for Karen, who realised that her mother would not support her
after she told her about her father's behaviour. For her both the abuse-related
and the disclosure-related events were stressful.[4] As an adolescent, Karen had to
continue to live with her father, who carried on sexually assaulting her siblings.
Not only was her disclosure as an adolescent traumatic but the court process was
extremely difficult to negotiate as well. Her mother stood by her father throughout the court case and behaved almost as if she didn't have children. However,
at least there was eventually a successful outcome which was not true for Tina.

Tina's story – 'groomed by the family'

Tina lived by the coast with her daughter. Her father died when she and her twin brother were babies. She was sexually assaulted by her aunt's boyfriend, a man in his sixties, from the age of eight until she was 16 when she threatened to tell on him. He would touch her genitals and masturbate. Tina never felt safe in his presence, even in a room full of people. She found out that he was molesting one of her female cousins, too. As she got older she became angrier and tried to defend herself by kicking him.

The worst betrayal happened when, as a mother herself, Tina wanted to protect her own daughter from this man. She repeatedly told family members what he had done to her, but they closed ranks and refused to do anything about it. As a result Tina ended up cutting off contact with her entire family which she found extremely painful. She eventually reported the abuse to the police, who decided not to prosecute as the victimiser was in his nineties by then. In many ways Tina felt that her family was the trap that she was caught in.

Tina was very tearful throughout the session and warned me before we started the interview that she would probably cry. However, she was highly motivated to tell her story. I felt very sad as I listened to what had happened to her as a young child and I admired the way she was choosing to protect her own daughter from her family.

> The reason that I'm here was my aunt's boyfriend instigated sexual activity with me when I was about eight. He was about 65 and he was a lot of fun. He had a boat and a panel van with a television, so we used to watch television as we were driving. And he had a fridge; we always had Fanta and lemonade. And he used to play games with us and he was always very free with money, giving us lollies and icy poles and things like that.
>
> The first time he touched me on the breasts and I was really shocked. I knew that he wasn't supposed to be touching me like that, but I didn't know what to do about it. I was really frightened that my aunt would be cranky with me and so I didn't say anything. He gave a lot of attention to me, which I loved because I didn't have that, because I didn't have a father. He was always trying to grab me and touch me. Even though I liked him and I thought he was fun, I didn't like it. And it had gone on for sort of a long time to me, so I thought I was a willing participant. So I thought, 'Oh, this is wrong and if I say anything I'm going to get in trouble.' So I didn't say anything to anyone.

I could hear that Tina blamed herself for what was happening to her. She knew it was wrong and she believed that many of her family members knew about it, but chose to turn a blind eye. This preserved the fantasy of the 'happy family'. No one was willing to confront the victimiser or her aunt with the unpalatable truth.

[After trying to tell] it didn't stop. It got worse. And he used to [crying] put his fingers inside me and masturbate behind me, and he would get all shaky and sort of dribble. And it was very frightening for me. This is a difficult thing to say but sometimes physically it was pleasurable but emotionally it was terrible. And I thought I was bad, that I was doing this with him. I felt I was doing it.

The whole family knew about it, but nobody did anything. My aunt was viewed as this delicate person and everyone thought that she was on the edge and that she would jump off a cliff. When I was 13 I was really angry and I would fight him off and kick him. But he was very clever. He was very adept. Even in a room full of people I wasn't safe. Anyway, he was trying to give me money to fly down and stay with them. And I thought, 'He's going to rape me if I go then.' I didn't want to go. And I said, 'If you don't take this money back, I will tell my aunt everything.' I knew that I was still keeping the secret within the family. And he never touched me again after that.

I think it had a lot of effect on me. I was very angry when I was a child, and when I was a teenager. I was furious with my mother and sister, and when I think back now, I think underneath it all it was about them not doing anything and not protecting me. When I was older I said to my sister, 'Don't you invite him. I don't want him near my daughter. He's a paedophile. He will sexually assault her. Don't invite him to this party.' And so they didn't. And then when my aunt said, 'Oh, they haven't invited him. Do you know why?' she said, 'Oh, it's just an oversight.' So the rest of the family just closed ranks.

Eventually, Tina decided that she needed to tell her aunt what was happening to her, for her own sanity. She described the pressure placed on her by other family members who didn't want her to destroy their image of their magical family. Although she was unable to confront her aunt with the truth, she eventually told the police who took no action because of the age of the victimiser by that stage.

I wanted to go and tell my aunt and we went down there, and I, and I got a lot of opposition from the family. Everyone told me I would kill her, I would destroy her, and I was selfish, and was going to ruin everybody's life. And when I got down there, I found I couldn't do it.

It took me two years to go to the police after that, because I just about had a nervous breakdown afterwards. It was pretty awful [crying]. It was like my whole family died in a car accident or a plane crash. It was very difficult. I'm talking about it now and it's very painful, but I don't live it in my normal life any more. But if I start talking about it then it's very painful. It's probably the family's betrayal is actually more painful than the actual. Oh, I don't know, it's hard to say. The assaults were awful, too. I suppose they were equally painful. I think it is worse that the family did what they did, and I've glossed over it but

> it was dreadful. They just didn't want to do anything about it. They wanted to keep the family intact. They wanted to play the perfect family, and still have the parties. And to me, it meant nothing, that's not family to me. So I think what happens in my family is that the rights of individuals is sort of removed for the good of the family. It's a bit like the family is the trap.

Tina recognised that her family operated as a form of honey trap for unsuspecting children, supported by adults who chose to turn a blind eye to what was going on in their midst. With a heavy heart, she eventually decided to have nothing to do with them and cut off all contact.

> In the end I said to my mother, 'That's it. Don't phone me, don't anything. Keep away from me.' And that was a very hard thing to do because my father had died and my brother was killed so I felt a lot of responsibility towards my mother. But I was going to end up in the psychiatric ward.

Tina was worried that her daughter would be lured back into the family system by the gifts and the attention that her family gave her. She was worried that the sexual abuse would continue into the next generation. This made taking a stand all the more important to her, in order to protect future generations of children from being sexually abused.

> Sometimes I have no energy. I miss the fun that we had and all the parties. I had a magical childhood in many ways, if only you could remove the sexual assault. I won't go to my mother's funeral when it happens. They won't be kind if I do. Making the break was very painful for me, intensely painful. I'm worried about my daughter. I would never forgive myself if she was sexually assaulted. She is pulled in by the family. It's almost like you are being groomed by the family. They keep on sending her $50 cheques and presents for her birthday. A little girl likes the attention. I'm not confident that she won't be drawn back in when she is older. And I also have my suspicions that her cousins may become perpetrators.

During the interview Tina weighed up the impact of the abuse against the impact of the loss of her family. In the end she decided that the betrayal by the family had been far worse than anything else. She felt that she had no choice other than to protect her own daughter and decided not to attend family functions with her victimiser. The family steadfastly refused to acknowledge that there was a problem and denied her account of events. In order to hold onto her own sanity and sense of reality, she decided to reject the family and pay the price. This decision had been painful to arrive at and painful to execute.

Strength of the survivor discourses for Tina

Although female socialisation still carries with it certain stereotypical expectations which can be oppressive, it also allows for greater acceptance of female victims. Perhaps this makes it socially easier for women, than for men, to talk about their maltreatment as children and to seek help. Paradoxically, it may enable more women to have more of a voice and to work through their experiences more openly, leading to better long-term adjustment than for male sexual abuse victims.[5] Women are also socialised to ask for support from others, and are perhaps more likely to benefit from being members of a group or community of fellow sufferers. Certainly, Tina had received some useful therapeutic support from various counsellors that helped her to make the decisions that she made to expose her victimiser and to protect her own daughter from these patterns of behaviour being repeated down the generations.

There are many variables that might impact on the decision as to whether or not to disclose abuse, including abuse severity, family environment and gender. One study suggested that women were more likely to disclose their abuse to others and to receive positive reactions to the disclosure than men.[6] However, it is not clear whether or not the women experienced more severe forms of child sexual abuse than the men. Tina certainly felt comfortable with the identity as a survivor and found it comforting to talk to other women about their experiences, and it is likely the socialisation process for women makes this easier than for men.[7] Women who join survivor groups tend to have good outcomes in adulthood in terms of self-esteem.[8] It is not clear whether this is as a consequence of their resiliency or influential in the development of resilience. By contrast, the inability to talk about emotional experiences that are so essential to identity may create severe disconnections in men's relationships. No men in this study had reported their victimisers to the police or taken them to court as had these three women.

Jane's story – 'protecting my twin'

Jane was an identical twin in her early forties. She was an attractive woman and a single mother who preferred to live alone. She had been sexually abused by her violent father from the age of eight to 16, when her parents separated. Jane's father was an ex-military man who terrorised the entire family. He was violent towards Jane's mother, towards whom Jane never felt any love. Jane blamed her for failing to protect her children and, at times, appeared to be angrier with her mother than with her abusive father.

However, it was her twin's suffering that upset Jane the most. Throughout most of the interview Jane only cried when mentioning her twin's pain, not her own. Jane tried to protect her and believed that, if her father was molesting her, he would not touch her twin. Later on she was distressed to discover that her twin had tried to tell their mother what was happening. This had resulted in her twin being physically assaulted by her father.

As an adult Jane made a report to the police and her father did go to jail for a few years. However, she remained frightened of him and of going out with men. Later she married and had two children. Now separated, she preferred to have affairs with married men which seemed safer to her. She was still frightened of her father and moved frequently in case he ever found her. This is Jane's story, which started with an opportunity taken by her father.

> My mother went into hospital and my father said, 'Each night that your mum's away, one of you will share my bed.' That's how it started with him touching me. And he was violent. One time we were five minutes late getting home, and he beat us. He used a fibreglass fishing rod that left cuts and welts on us. My mother was hit fairly often, but not as much as my father's second wife. We were always very scared of him. I can never remember ever feeling any love at all for him, and funnily enough I can't for my mother either. Maybe she just was never there for us. I think she had her own problems.
>
> It started round the age of eight. At nine we went to boarding school and, for us, that was just great. We had escaped from them and we just felt so free. We ran away to stop them from sending us back to our parents during the school holidays. We did actually end up going overseas, and there the abuse for me really took hold. He might wake me up really early and take me down the garden, or for a walk, and do things then. He'd force me to perform oral sex on him. And always, 'You mustn't tell anybody. It's our secret.' But there was a hint of violence behind that as well. A little bit later on, when I was around 12, 13, if I tried to get away he'd hold me by my hair, or hold me forcefully, or take it out on me in another way.

Jane's father was highly manipulative and demonstrated the grooming behaviour typical of paedophiles, as we saw with Karen. Initially, he told her that what they were doing was a secret, but later he used threats of violence to silence her. She endured severe beatings and sexual abuse, partly in the hope that she could protect her twin sister from harm.

> At the age of 13 he sort of pre-warned me that he was going to go all the way. He had penetrated me with his fingers and sure enough on my thirteenth birthday, he penetrated me, which I remember was painful. And I did bleed. And he said if I ever fell pregnant he would sort it out. This abuse was almost on a daily basis until I was 16, when my mother divorced him. He was having an affair with another woman, who he actually ended up marrying. But still I hadn't told anybody about it. I hadn't told a soul.

Jane told most of her story in a monotone and seemed quite detached from her feelings. But when she described how her twin sister had become involved and had been physically threatened by her father, she became highly distressed on her behalf. It was as if she wanted, above all, to protect her twin from any pain.

> We used to go to school late with tears streaming down our faces and bruises on us, and still no one at the school ever did anything. They used to just shake their heads and tut, tut, and say, 'Go to class.' Unbeknown to me my sister had tried to help. She had approached my mother and said, 'I think something's going on, because Dad comes in the room very early in the morning and I can hear the bed squeaking.' And my mother's reaction was 'There's nothing you can do about it.' After that he got my sister on her own at various times and threatened to kill her.

Jane hinted that her mother might have been sexually abused as a child. This might have partly explained her behaviour but did not excuse it in her eyes. Jane still felt angry and abandoned by her mother and oscillated between believing and not believing that her mother had known about the abuse. She described their complex relationship in which 'she knew that I knew that she knew, that this had been going on and that she'd done nothing'. One day her mother had slapped her out of frustration, as if in punishment for what she could not acknowledge was happening in the family.

> My mother would come into the room and start slapping me around. And she never said why she was slapping me around the face, and being horrible. But I knew that she knew that I knew why she was doing it. But even to this day she's never turned round and said sorry or 'I should have been there for you.'

Like Karen, Jane chose to believe that she was a virgin when she had sexual intercourse with someone of her own age for the first time. She was very frightened of sexual intimacy and went to great lengths to avoid it as a young adult.

> When I was probably 16, I remember the first sexual experience being then and I was having a period and there was a bit of blood, and the guy thought I was a virgin and I thought, 'Oh well, maybe I could pretend that is the first time.' I remember round about the age of 19 when guys used to come calling to take me out, I'd like go into hyperventilating and I'd go and hide in cupboards and hope they'd go away. I suppose it comes from having tried to hide myself, to get away from my father.

Although as an adult Jane reported her father to the police, she was very cynical about the impact that this had on his life. She didn't believe that it impacted on him a great deal if at all.

My father married this lady and she lost a baby while she was pregnant through being beaten up. She lost teeth. Then we heard that his stepdaughter age 12 was very upset and crying. I thought I can't allow somebody else to go through it, so I reported him to the police. And he did go to jail for a short time, but as far as I'm concerned it didn't make any difference at all. It may have just tarnished his reputation, but it didn't stop his abuse. I didn't want anything to do with him. I lost even more respect for my mother, in not trying to help that girl, after I'd finally got round to telling her when I was 18. That was the first time I told anybody, because I was starting to like break down, hiding behind doors just crying.

I think it upsets me more, not the fact that I was abused but the fact that it's really messed up, not just my life, but my twin's life. We'd never said anything to each other. That could have been a way of protecting each other. I didn't even ask her if it was happening to her. I would never have been strong enough to commit suicide and leave her, because it would have meant that she would have been maybe the next victim. If he was doing it to me, he wouldn't be doing it to her. My twin and I had a big fight recently. Funnily enough, it is more upsetting to me that my twin [starts crying] has suffered so much as well. We're talking a lot more now after our big blow out, but we still can't really talk about what happened. We did at one stage, but I haven't told her half of even what I've just told you now.

Having had her own daughter, Jane felt a tremendous bond of love and a strong desire to protect her from harm. She then found it impossible to understand why her own mother had done nothing to stop the abuse. Her own mother's non-protective behaviour weighed more heavily on her than her father's abusive behaviour, and drove her desire to speak out and prevent future sexual abuse of children.

I have a daughter and I just had such a strong bond with her [crying], and I just can't understand my mother not having that same bond with us. But I do find that I watch my daughter. I try not to overreact, I let her go to sleepovers, but I sort of watch for signs with the parents, especially the father.

Sadly, Jane had never talked to her twin about the sexual abuse. She had never asked her twin if she had been sexually abused. She couldn't work out why she had been singled out by their father. She remained highly protective of her twin as an adult, and felt her twin's pain very acutely. Having interviewed so many people where the father had sexually abused all his children in turn, I couldn't help being concerned that Jane's twin might also have been sexually abused by her father and that Jane might, one day, find this out. I sincerely hoped that this suspicion was wrong as this would add to Jane's pain.

Jane's vulnerability to mental health problems

Jane certainly suffered at the hands of her ruthless father and her ineffectual mother and appeared to demonstrate some symptoms of dissociation and depression. At first reading, most studies appear to suggest that women who have had abusive childhood sexual experiences with adults go on to develop more severe mental health problems than men. However, on closer inspection, this appears be an oversimplification since the women studied have usually experienced more severe or more recent forms of abuse, including physical abuse, than the men interviewed. Thus the higher level of adult psychopathology among women may be explained by the severity of the abuse they experienced, as was the case with Jane, and not by their gender. It is possible that women actually cope better on average with childhood adversity than men.[9]

NARRATIVE OF JUSTICE AT ANY COST

Karen, Tina and Jane told a *narrative of justice at any cost*. Despite being groomed as young children, being severely physically and sexually abused, and being fearful for their lives, they emerged from childhood stronger women as a result. They believed that they had been transformed as a consequence of their experiences. They saw themselves as survivors and felt good about the way they had overcome the hardships of the past. In particular, they felt good about the way they had been able to protect other children from harm by reporting their victimisers to the police. As a consequence of making a report, they had eventually felt the need to cut off from their families who supported the victimisers. They were unwilling to risk the abuse continuing into the next generation. These actions helped them to develop a powerful sense of themselves as seeking justice, breaking the cycle and preventing future sexual abuse. Unlike Jewels, Emm and Heather, who chose to remain silent in order to protect other people, these three women chose to speak out about their childhood maltreatment in order to prevent future suffering.

These women gave the clearest descriptions of being groomed by their victimisers. For Karen and Tina, their experiences were in some ways pleasurable to begin with – either physically or emotionally. At first Karen was told by her father that what was happening was a special secret between them, and Tina was given lollies and treats by her aunt's boyfriend. As time went by, the mood changed and they were threatened with violence or punishment if they resisted. Jane's father was violent with her from the beginning. Like Karen, she was far too frightened of her father to risk his anger by telling anyone what he was doing to her. She knew all too well what he was capable of doing. Tina described the grooming process as a collective effort, since everyone wanted to maintain the status quo and the illusion of a 'happy family' who had lots of fun together. She was fearful that her own daughter was being seduced by the family, with gifts and invitations to join in the fun.

Karen and Tina both tried to tell their mothers what had happened to them when they were children. When little changed as a result, they still had to continue to live with the situation and push away all thoughts of what had happened to them. Jane did not try to tell overtly but, from her description, it should have been obvious to the adults in her life what was happening to her. Trying to tell as children and not being believed may have fuelled the anger felt by these women about the injustice of their situations. Karen and Tina felt severely let down by their families and by their mothers, in particular, for failing to do anything to change the situation and to keep them safe from further harm. Jane felt angry that someone had not recognised what was happening and intervened in the situation. These early incidents increased their resolve to tell the police as adults and to seek justice.

The act of standing up to their victimisers and reporting them to authorities empowered these women, even though it came at considerable personal cost. It enabled them to feel proud of themselves for taking action to protect future generations of children. The cost had been the fracturing of their relationships with other family members, often beyond repair. It was very important to these women to tell someone outside the family and to receive validation of their childhood experiences. They went to the police against the wishes of their families and demonstrated great courage in facing and overcoming the challenges that they experienced in their personal lives, as a result of both their incestuous experiences and the consequences of making a police report.

Although suicidality was no longer a problem for these three women, they had faced extremely difficult periods in their lives when they had found it necessary to cut off all contact with members of their family. Karen and Tina both reported feeling intense pain and anger about what they saw as a betrayal by their families. All three women believed that their sexual relationships and their intimate lives had been affected by their childhood experiences.

Having acknowledged the impact of abuse, the overwhelming message from these women was that they had the courage to stand up to the abuse, make a report to the police and break the cycle for future generations. They took pride in their achievements, despite the devastating consequences in terms of the loss of connection with their families and the impact of their intimate relationships.

In the next chapter, five men and women describe how they refused to be defined by their childhood experiences. They, too, recognised the impact of their childhood experiences but refused to be seen as victims, or even as survivors. They had developed spiritually and wanted to be seen as people, rather than be defined by their histories.

SUMMARY

Key points

- These three women told a *narrative of justice at any cost.*
- They demonstrated remarkable resilience when facing enormous challenges. They overcame their incestuous childhood experiences and, as adults, accepted the consequences of reporting family members to the police.
- They believed that they had been severely affected by their incestuous experiences and wanted to protect other children from such experiences.
- They tried to tell someone as children but were not believed. This may have fuelled their anger and their resolve to seek justice as adults.
- These women describe being transformed by their childhood adversity and gaining the strength to stand up to their victimisers.
- They paid a considerable personal cost in that they were obliged to cut off all contact with their families.

CHAPTER 8

Remaining defiant

INTRODUCTION

> **Chapter aims**
> - Tell the narratives of five men and women who were *remaining defiant* and refusing to be defined by their childhood sexual experiences.
> - Explore the coping mechanisms they used in their dysfunctional families and their need to feel normal.
> - Describe how they overcame the profound impact that their experiences had on them.
> - Outline how they grew spiritually and transcended their experiences, and didn't want to be stereotyped as a result of their childhood maltreatment.

Five men and women did not want their identities to be linked to their childhood experiences which they believed they had transcended. They were more than the sum of these experiences and wanted to be recognised as such. This was a defiant narrative in many ways. Belinda described this feeling in the following words: 'I don't feel sort of trapped by it any more. Like it's not the only thing that defines who I am any more, and that there's so much more to life than that.'

Diana, Belinda, Norm and Will had several sexual experiences as young children whereas Rod's experience happened only once. They had all been brought up in families where physical and emotional abuse was commonplace. The main link between them was the almost defiant way in which they refused to be defined by these experiences. Most reacted with anger and aggression as adolescents and young adults. They had many difficulties in their adult lives which they attributed to their childhood sexual experiences. However, they had overcome these problems, usually with little help from professionals, and believed that they had grown spiritually as a result of their experiences.

In some ways there were similarities between this group and those who had broken silence recently about their experiences. Many were men who had chosen not to think or talk about their experiences and believed that they had moved beyond them. The main difference was that those telling a *narrative of a silence recently broken* believed that their childhood sexual experiences had no real impact on their lives, except perhaps sexually, whereas these men and women knew that they had been affected by their experiences but believed that they had overcome these difficulties and refused to be stereotyped as a result.

REFUSING TO BE DEFINED BY CHILDHOOD SEXUAL EXPERIENCES

The main characteristic of those telling this narrative was that they refused to have their identities linked to their childhood maltreatment. They were fully aware of the impact that these experiences had had on their lives, but they rejected the way that society tried to label them as either victims or survivors.

Diana's story – 'I'd rather be seen as a tart than a victim'

Diana was a woman in her early fifties who had worked mainly in the helping professions. She had grown up with a violent, alcoholic father. She was his favourite and took on the role of protector of her sisters, persuading her father not to hurt them. As a small child Diana was touched sexually by various men. At the age of 14 she was pack-raped by 14 men. This experience was followed a few weeks later by another violent rape. She didn't tell her parents for fear that it would distress her mother and that her father would end up in jail for killing someone.

Diana decided she needed a man for protection, even though she despised them. She met her current partner when she was 19 and worked through a lot of physical, sexual and emotional issues in this relationship. Diana believed that the two rapes had a big impact on her. She became violent and angry as a young woman, luring men into sexually compromising positions with the intent of physically harming them, in order to even the score. As an adult she was grateful that she had never managed to hurt anyone seriously, or get herself reported to the police. She also used drugs and alcohol to excess and had sex with both men and women, even though she now identifies as heterosexual.

In her thirties Diana became a born-again Christian and worked with prisoners, sexual offenders, alcoholics and drug abusers. She showed a remarkable empathy for her rapists and when she met one of them in jail, she was able to forgive him. Diana was a great raconteur and a forceful character, which comes across in her story which is almost humorous at times.

> Secrets are strange things, what gets kept a secret and what gets talked about. When you come from a family where there's alcoholism and domestic violence, you're brought up with secrets, because everyone has to believe that you're

a normal family and nobody hurts anybody, and you're loved, and you get milk and cookies when you come home [said ironically]. My father wanted a boy and so I've always been the tomboy. He bashes the entire family up, but he doesn't touch me. I'm the golden child. I'm possum pie. But everyone else in the family, they all get bashed. I'm the one that stops him from bashing everyone.

There's not a lot that I do actually remember about the rape. I don't push myself to recall because I can't see a purpose in the recollection of it. The first part was terrifying because you're fearful for your life. As you get further into a pack rape, it takes so long that your panic and your fear diminishes, because you're still alive, so you think, 'They're not going to kill me.'

As Diana told her story, I could imagine her as a young girl working out that she was in grave danger. She knew that she had to hide her fear from these violent men and she took whatever power she could, even in such a desperate situation. Her ability to empathise with the young men who raped her was truly remarkable. She described what happened half-way through the pack rape.

And there was an Italian boy, these are kids, they ranged from 13 to about 25. This crucifix on this very long chain was slapping me in the face and I started to laugh at the irony of this. And I suddenly realised that this boy lost his erection [clicks her fingers], quick as a flash, gone. So I thought, in amongst all this, I have power, the power of the cunt. In that moment I didn't see myself as the victim. I saw myself as being in a position of power.

I suspect that there were some there that were virgins. I used to worry for those boys. I used to think how hideous for their very, very first time, that they would have an experience with a woman like that. I felt for them. They all went to jail, not through anything I did, but they were eventually arrested because they kept on raping women.

Just as Diana's violent upbringing helped her to survive being raped, it also taught her to keep secrets. She chose to protect her mother from knowing about the rape, because she believed that her mother would blame herself.

I don't want my parents to know about this. My father would be in jail for murder, if he found out about this. My mother, it would kill her. She would never, ever recover. They may as well have raped her. And to this day, my mother, I've never, ever told her. And I'm very, very close with my mother; I ring her almost every day. But I would never, ever tell her this story because she wouldn't cope with it. She would see herself as in some way responsible, and it happened because she was a bad mother. But that was not the case. It happened because I was a disobedient child.

Anyway, the second rape was a really violent rape [voice darkens], savage and angry, and a power rape. After that I decided I had to have a boyfriend, to stop getting raped all the time. The men all respected the other men, but they don't respect the women. But if the man had a woman, well you don't touch that woman, not out of respect for her, out of respect for *him*. So I got a boyfriend but then I got pregnant. By this stage I was 15. By 18 I was really dangerous. I should have been having counselling, intensive therapy. I used to carry a knife, I used to stab men. I used to lure men into situations where I could stab them, on the promise of sex, get them into dark places and run them through with a knife. I never killed anyone, which amazes me.

This is a remarkable story of transcending a terrifying experience. Diana was severely damaged by being raped. She became an angry young woman, behaving in a dangerous way to seek revenge. I wondered if she had come to view men as objects, in the way that they had objectified her so brutally. Although she identified as heterosexual and had a long-term male partner, she had relationships with women as well and seemed confused about her sexuality. She struggled to work out what had caused these complications in her intimate life: being raped; being a lesbian; or being with the wrong male partner.

I could not cope at all with the idea of marriage. And that was purely through my mother's indoctrination. Because of her marriage, she used to constantly say, 'Diana, don't get married. Don't let them own you. No man should own another person and that's all marriage is, so don't fall for it.' So I never did. I really despised men and saw men as a means to an end.

I don't really know whether it was a consequence of those events, but I was a homosexual for probably 15 years and still, to this day, feel like I'm a homosexual that lives a heterosexual lifestyle [laughs]. I could never really work out whether my sexual orientation was a genetic issue, a hormone issue, a by-product of circumstances that repulsed me from men, or what it was. Am I like this because all those things happened to me? Or am I like this because it's just my orientation and I would have been like this whether those things happened or not? Or am I like this because maybe I'm with the wrong partner and I should find either a male or a female that makes me happy?

It was seven years before Diana could have sex with a man without crying. She was also afflicted by many physical illnesses that she associated with the rapes, as well as alcohol-related health problems. It is amazing to me that she overcame the profound consequences on her physical health and on her desire to have sexual intercourse.

Quite often I would have sex and I would vomit. It would just nauseate me to the pit of my stomach. And I mean that's a pretty horrible, right in the middle of having sex with someone and all you can do is just heave your guts up. That's hard on your partner. 'What – I make you sick? I literally make you ill. No, I don't want to have sex with you if I'm going to make you vomit every time.' Then I developed a reaction against sperm, and that was all psychosomatic. The body smell of a man was repulsive to me. The smell of sperm would make me just vomit, and that's from being forced to have oral sex.

Diana experienced many of the difficulties in adulthood that we have come to associate with childhood sexual assault, including drug and alcohol problems. Interestingly, she did not believe that talking about either of the rapes or pushing herself to remember what had happened was a helpful thing for her to do. She believed in the healing power of love but did not expect to receive such a gift from a counsellor.

I did have a six-month period there where I was abusing a lot of drugs, mainly marijuana and alcohol. Now I'm a teetotaller. I was about 34 and I had a series of strokes, brought about as a reaction to the alcohol. I've smoked marijuana for about 30 years, I'm a regular smoker.

[I have] no faith in counsellors. No faith in the system, any system. If ever I discussed it with anyone it was usually for the purposes of cathartic purposes, therapeutic purposes in relationship to someone else's healing. If it didn't have a purpose, then there was no reason to talk about it, to my mind. When it comes down to healing, well, love heals all. And you can't really expect your counsellor to love you.

Diana's empathy for some of her rapists

Some survivors of child sexual abuse are able to avoid blaming themselves for their experiences by attributing events either to their abusers' personalities (e.g. sadistic traits, evil personalities or mental illness) or to their circumstances, rather than to themselves.[1] This was true for Diana who recognised that some of her rapists were, indeed, evil. However, when she became a born-again Christian and experienced God's forgiveness, Diana was grateful to her God for giving her such experiences. She believed that her horrendous childhood experiences had made her stronger. 'I wouldn't change any of that, because it made me a strong woman.'

Remarkably, Diana was able to show empathy for some of her rapists, because she believed that they had also been damaged as a result of the experience. She saw the younger rapists as victims who ended up paying for their crimes. As an adult she met one of her rapists, when she was working at a jail. Diana had been praying for a sign from her God that she knew how to forgive. Happily for her, she felt able to forgive him and felt blessed as a result. She was a feisty woman and summed up her views by saying: 'You know, I'd rather be seen as a tart than a victim.' This view was echoed by Belinda who also rejected, being labelled as a victim or a survivor.

Belinda's story – 'a hole in your soul'

Belinda was an impressive young woman in her late twenties who, despite recent surgery, was determined to be interviewed. She was brought up on a rural property with her mother, her alcoholic stepfather whom she called 'Dad' and her stepsister. Her biological father left when she was a baby. Belinda's stepfather sexually abused her from the age of five to 13. Her stepmother and father eventually found out and reported him to the police. The sexual abuse stopped, but Belinda had to continue to live with her victimiser. Indeed, her mother and stepsister are still living with him now.

Belinda felt that, as an adult, she had made massive strides to overcome a problem that had overwhelmed her for so many years. She worried that her stepfather might have hurt other children, too, and was concerned that she hadn't done enough to stop him as a child. However, she also felt resentful that she was expected to carry this additional burden of responsibility alone. She started to tell her story with a haunting image of a small child, walking to school, worrying that there was something wrong with her.

> I just remember walking to primary school and thinking, 'What's wrong with me? Why doesn't my Dad love me?' And 'Why aren't I good enough?' I just wanted him to be proud of me. I knew something wasn't how it should be with the whole father–daughter relationship. And I just didn't feel that love and care, it wasn't there. It's a bit of a hole in your soul, when you kind of miss out on just being allowed to be a kid, and being accepted that way.
>
> Mum got married, had me, and then she was divorced and I didn't know my real dad until I was seven. When I was two, she remarried and had a daughter. There were lots of issues around my stepfather besides abuse because he was alcoholic, angry and name-calling, and pointing out the differences between me and my sister, saying we weren't real sisters. It was 'divide and conquer'; he was isolating me within the family, from early on.
>
> I can't remember when the abuse started but it escalated and escalated. We moved interstate and it got worse and worse. Mum was working night-shifts, so there wasn't really anywhere to go. We had a small acreage, but it was eight kilometres to town, so there was no running away. And I had this little sister. I thought, 'If I do go anywhere or kick up any kind of stink, she would be the next target.' I just felt like I jinxed whatever relationships that anyone had around me. I was going to wreck them just because I was alive. He used to say I was a home-wrecker and that I was trying to make his life difficult or miserable. I was scared of rocking the family boat. And it's not really fair for my sister to

suddenly lose a dad. All I ever wanted was a dad, and so I didn't want her to not have that.

Clearly, her stepfather was a highly manipulative man who put her into an impossible position. When Belinda's stepmother worked out what was going on and went to the police, Belinda was manipulated into saying very little for fear that she would cause the breakdown of another marriage.

> I was visiting my real dad and his wife and she figured out something was wrong. And Mum had the biggest shock of her life, with this angry phone call from my real dad, because she didn't have a clue what was going on. And everybody was upset. I had to talk to police and the department. Just the embarrassment, worrying about what people would think of me, not wanting to hurt my mum and my sister, fear of the unknown.
>
> I hardly said anything at all to the police, because I just didn't trust anybody. I basically told people the minimum of what I thought they wanted to hear, to get them off my back. Just things like 'He made me touch his penis,' which was all true anyway, but not the rest of what happened. I felt really in the spotlight and uncomfortable, and the police came to the school, and made me talk about it in front of the principal. They were asking me about going to court, so I said, 'No way. Get lost and leave me alone.'
>
> So it never went to court. Nothing ever happened except that he stopped doing it out of fear, embarrassment. He didn't have to not live with us. Nothing happened. It was never mentioned again like anywhere, by anyone until recently, when I got really depressed and suicidal, and I ended up going on antidepressants and getting counselling.
>
> I started trying to tell my mother how it was affecting my life. And she doesn't really get it, that it still affects me. Sometimes I think even I don't know what happened, but then I have a lot of these flashbacks and I know it happened.

Belinda suffered from depression as a young adult and often felt suicidal. She also had sleeping problems and difficulties in her intimate life. These are not uncommon difficulties to have as a direct result of incestuous experiences in childhood. She was angry that her mother continued to play happy families and pretend that nothing had happened to her, and that she got to carry the responsibility by herself and to suffer alone.

> Mum was asking me do I want him to leave? To ask me that I don't think was really fair. I was just so worried about everybody else and I'd been told I was a home wrecker. And Mum would be really upset. So of course I said, 'No, no.' Somehow I'd ended up feeling all that responsibility for the whole family, and

even for my mother's relationships. I just remember him on the steps crying, saying, 'Do you forgive me?' And of course I had to say yes. You're supposed to love your dad and honour your parents.

I've just had to carry all this emptiness and all these emotions, and everyone else was just allowed to go on pretending everything was just fine. And they still are. They're all still living together in the same house, like they're a family and I still feel the isolated one. It's been really hard that way, to sort of feel close to my sister and my mum. There was always this lingering question of 'Well, should I pursue something legally now?' I'm thinking, 'Well, what if there was other people?' Even if it was like the minutest possibility. Now I do feel worried and scared and guilty about that, for not doing more as a kid [with frustration in her voice].

Belinda described how she had developed sleeping problems and had difficulties relaxing in bed at night. As a child she had deliberately tried to stay awake in the vain hope that she could somehow avoid her stepfather's sexual abuse. She found it hard to be sexual with men, since she felt little or no sexual desire. She recognised that this was a problem in her relationships.

I can't even have a normal relationship, like I have no desire to have sex or anything like that. So that's obviously been a big deal with my relationships. It seems like the only person who was really lastingly affected was me. Every time I went to bed it was like 'Stay awake, stay awake, I've got to stay awake.' So now when I go to bed, I can't relax. I just felt if I had some kind of warning that he was coming, I could somehow do something to make it not happen, without endangering my sister.

Belinda was sustained by her faith. She was in the process of overcoming her past and becoming fulfilled as a person. She didn't want to end the interview on a negative note and wanted everyone to know that she no longer felt defined by what had happened to her as a child. Just before the interview, she had organised a public meeting within her church community on the topic of child sexual abuse and she felt proud that she had been able to stand up and talk about her experiences. She hoped that people within that community would think no less of her for being so open, although she knew that she was taking a risk. However, she expected people to continue to respect her.

The most helpful thing has probably been my faith in God, actually. Even though I might never make sense of it, or I might always have that real sad feeling inside, I don't feel trapped by it any more. It's not the only thing that defines who I am any more, and there's so much more to life than that. For 20 years my whole life has been defined by that, and living around that, and now I can see past it into something else, which is really, really great, and really hopeful. It makes me feel like I respect myself a lot more by being able to say that I was sexually abused as a child, and I don't expect you to think any less of me as a person, or to judge me, or to think that I might become a perpetrator or anything like that.

Belinda's rejection of the survivor discourse

Belinda rejected the social identity as a survivor because it anchors women's sense of themselves in their abuse. She thought that this was too stigmatising. To be a survivor, you need to have survived something and be willing to speak out about what has happened to you. For some women, this is a useful thing to do as it helps them to feel a sense of solidarity with other survivors and to feel empowered to prevent future sexual abuse of children. For other women, it is daunting and potentially stigmatising to identify themselves as survivors and to speak out about their childhood maltreatment. It opens them up to being described as damaged goods and to being looked down on by others.

Although Belinda was willing to speak out about her experiences within her church community, she knew that she was taking a risk in doing so. She was aware that some people might try to stereotype her as a victim or survivor and not see her as a whole person. She explained that her abuse no longer defined her as a person. She was bigger than the sum of her history of sexual abuse and did not wish to be defined in this way.

The fact that Belinda's mother had been unable to support her daughter when the sexual abuse came out into the open and continues to live with her victimiser to this day also made disclosure difficult for Belinda. Unfortunately, this pattern of lack of family support is all too common. It is hard for children to disclose something that they don't fully understand but know to be culturally taboo and private in nature.[2] There is a need for the adult to provide a supportive structure, in order for the child to be able to make a disclosure.[3] Of course, it is also common for the non-offending parent to feel ambivalent following a disclosure of incest, even though this response is obviously not helpful to the child.[4] Children, such as Belinda, are sensitive to the responses of family members and disclosure can be a traumatic experience for them. Her disclosure had no real impact on the situation and Norm didn't even attempt to tell anyone for the same reason.

Norm's story – 'my pin-up girl'

Norm was a tall man with an imposing presence. In my clinical experience I had spoken to men who had revealed that they had been sexually abused as children by older men, but I was somewhat taken by surprise when he told me of his incestuous experiences with his mother. Somehow I wasn't mentally prepared for this.

Norm was in his early fifties and was a caregiver for his wife who had a chronic illness. They had chosen not to have children. Norm had a complex relationship with his alcoholic mother, who had worked as a prostitute. He would accompany her and her partner when they went out for the evening. Norm frequently saw his mother having sex with her clients. His feelings towards her became very confused as he grew older. He felt sexually attracted towards her and confused by her changeable responses to him.

Norm found it painful to remember these events and to talk about them. He became troubled in adolescence and was sent to boarding school. He described how one of his teachers had tried to help him. Despite this support, Norm was expelled from school aged 15 and started to use drugs and alcohol excessively. He had a number of satisfying homosexual experiences but identified as heterosexual. However, every woman that Norm met reminded him of his mother and he took out his anger and frustration with her on them. On her deathbed, he hoped for reconciliation, but this did not occur.

I found this interview challenging in two ways. First, it was not easy for Norm to tell his story. He spoke slowly and deliberately, as if he was remembering events and re-experiencing them in the room. He became so absorbed in the process that whenever the tape recorder clicked off, he was startled by the sound. He seemed to be in an almost trancelike state. Second, it was not easy for me to listen and I was aware of becoming very still, almost invisible, so as not to intrude on his memories. I felt shocked and saddened by what I heard, but I didn't want my facial expression or body posture to convey this to him. As a mother myself, my heart went out to the young boy he was describing. This is Norm's story in his own words.

> My mother was a call girl. Whenever I'd come home, there was always a string of uncles. One, in particular, who was very wealthy – millionaire – was pretty madly in love with my mother. He was also an alcoholic. My mother was an alcoholic, a blackout drinker. To this day, I'm pretty much convinced that a lot of things that she did she was completely unaware of. And having been a blackout drinker myself, I can appreciate that.
>
> I was like Little Lord Fauntleroy, I had suits, double-breasted blazers. And I would go out with them. They'd start off in the more posh places in town, and end up in a blood and guts bar at four in the morning. I became a kind of lure for other people. Most of the time it was a kind of a pleasant experience, being with my mother [in bed]. But there were other times when it was very smothering, very clutching. And there were times when she didn't have any clothes on and I didn't have any clothes on. I really didn't like that feeling, wet, hot, sweaty contact with her.

Some incidents stood out in his mind as particularly humiliating and confusing.

He learned various forms of escape as a child, including a form of dissociation[5] which he describes here.

> One night Greg decided that I needed to be spanked, and they had me take all my clothes off. And they were both naked. He didn't really hurt me but it was more like a shaming thing, one being naked in front of him, and then wondering what I'd done wrong. Then my mother embraced me and snuggled me in her breasts and told me to go to sleep. Greg had an erection through the whole thing. And then they just had sex and I couldn't sleep so I had to pretend to be asleep. And that was actually a pattern that went on for a few years, just pretending not to be there. And I used to be able to, I guess it's a form of dissociation, but just make myself really small or I made the environment I was in very large. It's like to go to that lamp [points at light across room] would take five light years.

Norm described a kaleidoscope of memories, not making sense all the time. It was as if he was being flooded by memories and didn't know how to put them into narrative form.

> My mother became my pin-up girl. And there's this one time, my mother is just there spread-eagled on the bed, naked. She wakes up and starts screaming at me that I'm a pervert. It's really confusing, because there've been levels of sexual intimacy that had taken place before then. I have no real sense of right or wrong around this. I mean it's exciting, it's dangerous. And I think I learned to just not talk about any of this stuff. I'm not really talking too much about it right now. I mean I have memories of touching my mother, but not penetrating her, certainly kissing her and even French kissing her. I used to get a hard on.
>
> At boarding school there was a lot of homosexuality, not only amongst the clergy but the whole choir thing. We'd go to the choir master's apartment and he'd let us drink. And there'd be a lot of horsing around. I was fascinated by paintings like 'The rape of the Sabine women' so I used to do a lot of drawings of mutilated women. And the science teacher ended up with these drawings. And he's actually one of the first of a group of compassionate people that came into my life. I didn't tell him too much, but I think I told him enough so that he kept an eye out on me. Eventually, I got in too much trouble and he couldn't do anything, and I was expelled.

Norm knew that his sexual behaviour in adulthood had been influenced by what happened to him as a child. He had a complicated love–hate relationship with his mother until her death.

> I have had a number of homosexual experiences. But I used to think a lot about

my mother and I used to dress up like my mother sometimes, put her clothes on, masturbate. When she had guests I would listen, spy if I could, sort of became a peeping Tom. Anything I could do to arouse images. Throughout my life she'd remind me of my birth and how I'd destroyed her, how my conception and birth destroyed her future. I had no idea what it was like to live in a family, and whenever I'd be invited to a real family, it was such a treat to sit around a table at dinner and talk about what happened in the day.

In adolescence Norm was violent towards both men and women. Most of the women he met reminded him of his mother and he took out his anger and rage against her on them. His impulsive behaviour affected his ability to develop mature relationships with women in particular. He did many self-destructive things such as taking drugs, using alcohol to excess, stealing, having ultimately unrewarding sexual experiences and hurting the people closest to him.

I actually started to be sexually active, but it was very confusing in the beginning. And I found myself always running into my mother, whoever the woman was. A lot of the relationships that I've had have had the anger that I would have liked to have directed towards my mother, towards the women. I just didn't have a clue what I was doing.

I was also taking drugs. I became addicted to heroin for a while. I sort of became a hustler, I say 'sort of' because I actually didn't go very far sexually. I would just get in there and slip them a pill and steal stuff and go. Whenever I came back home, I'd look down in the courtyard to see if my mother was there, because she was always talking about killing herself. I mean emotional blackmail was just very high. And I've seen how I use it. And you know I just see a lot of the things that my mother did, I've repeated until I've become aware of it. I was angry with the hypocrisy, double standards, defending my mother when she got into trouble, taking care of my mother when she got into trouble. You know I guess anger that nobody [raising his voice] nobody did anything.

Norm's story didn't have a fairytale ending. In fact it ended bitterly.

And about a month before she died, she called me and told me she was sober. And we started spending some time together. And then she told me that she was sick, cancer, an operation, and then her physiognomy changed totally. And she had an infection and died. And one of the last things that she said to me was 'You're gutless'.

I knew that the interview had been a painful process of remembering for Norm. I phoned him afterwards and he told me that he felt 'empty, sad, relieved, concerned, alone, angry'. The only positive for him was that talking about it all reminded him that he still had unfinished business that he needed to work through. This interview affected me profoundly at the time, and I am moved whenever I reread it. My heart goes out to that little boy, particularly because the victimiser was his mother.

The profound impact of Norm's incestuous experiences

Even though we know that child sexual abuse is common among boys as well as girls and that many victimisers are women, there is still a tendency for victimhood to be constructed as something that happens to women and young girls. It is still a gendered discourse.[6] Victims of child sexual abuse are assumed to be female and victimisers assumed to be male. This gendered discourse is slowly being challenged. However, the meaning that men and women attribute to childhood sexual experiences has inevitably been influenced by these societal and cultural beliefs.

I, myself, was influenced by this belief. Even though I knew that mothers sexually abuse their sons, I still found it shocking to hear Norm's first-hand account of incest between a mother and son. I could understand his desire to be invisible, not to exist. I could understand his desire for revenge against women. I could understand the descent into drugs, alcohol, promiscuity and crime as an escape from painful reality. I admired Norm's resilience in the face of adversity. He worked through his own healing journey in therapy. He became sober through Alcoholics Anonymous, trained as a therapist, and was working to help others heal their own childhood wounds. Rod was still finding his way.

Rod's story – 'in solitary confinement'

Rod was an unemployed, single man in his late forties, living in a small country town. He had had a difficult childhood. His father left when he was a baby. His mother had contacts with the criminal world and had several partners. Rod was brought up by his aunt, whom he described as like a drill sergeant. When he was 11, a friend of his mother's boyfriend interfered with him.

Rod was full of shame and anger when he realised what had happened to him, and developed a strong hatred of gay men. He joined a skinhead gang and got into fights with homosexuals. Later he joined a bikie gang and became a heavy drinker. His sexual relationship with women never lasted for longer than a weekend.

> I was 11 or 12, and a friend had come to stay, and I knew nothing of homosexuality or paedophiles, or anything of that. I was pretty naive at that age. And this man was staying in my room downstairs. My mum and stepfather were living upstairs. He basically took advantage of me, being very friendly, seduced me, but I really didn't understand what had happened. He just sort of molested

me, had oral sex with me. And, from that time on, it's had a huge effect on my life, like both physically and mentally, psychologically.

I was intrigued because many things happened in Rod's childhood but he placed great significance on this particular sexual experience at the age of 11. He talked about losing his manhood, which he found extremely distressing. It was as if he felt that, by being seduced by a man, he had lost his ability to 'conquer' women and to become a man himself. He felt a great sense of hatred towards homosexual men as a result, since he equated paedophilia with homosexuality.[7] He joined a racist gang in which violence was endemic, and set about taking revenge for what had happened to him as a child.

As I grew to my mid-teens and understood what had happened at that time of him taking my manhood away from me, I began to get the sense of embarrassment, shame, guilt, and kept it to myself. And a sense of extreme rage and of hatred towards people like that. That's where I got involved with a gang of skinheads, and went deliberately looking for gay people to pay back for what had happened to me. At times [I] became very violent, losing control. And even the guys had no idea why I was so violent towards homosexual people, whereas they were sort of beating up Asians, coloured people etcetera, etcetera. A good percentage of homosexual people have come from abused backgrounds themselves and have gone that way, whereas I've gone the opposite way and vented all that anger and that rage upon them, when really they were not to blame.

I didn't tell Mum for fear of she wouldn't believe me, or 'He's not like that' and of it being spread out to other family members, and what their reactions would be. I kept it to myself because I had a great fear of being branded as gay myself, a fear of name calling. I shared it with no one. I just kept it locked away inside of me and I started drinking, 'cos I thought, well, that's all part and parcel of being an Aussie male. And it affected my relationships with males. I'd draw a line; no one would get close to me, not even women.

Rod described how his aggression was often fuelled by excessive alcohol. He seemed to link alcohol, sex and violence together. When he drank excessively he would want to have sex with a woman and, if she refused, would become violent towards her. He tried to fit in by behaving like a typical 'Aussie male', i.e. a heavy-drinking bloke who viewed women as sex objects. He was unable to trust anyone, particularly if they wanted to get close to him. He felt the need to keep people at a distance, so he isolated himself and kept his feelings well hidden.

In some ways, starting drinking was a way of suppressing those feelings. But the more a person drank, it was also a trigger. So in one way I was trying to desensitise myself to those feelings, in another way it was also a trigger of releasing that rage. I was always very abusive to my friends or people round about me. And especially women, I was always very abusive and wanted to lash out, in wanting to basically have sex with them. And if I didn't, wanting to pound the crap out of them.

I had a stereo image in my mind of what an Aussie male was. 'Big boys don't cry. Be the muncho [sic] man. Someone knocks you down, you get up. You express no emotional feeling whatsoever, not even when you're with a woman.' I saw women as sexual objects, to be used and abused, because that's how I saw the role models within my family and friends. 'Monkey see, monkey do.' And so I imitated that and all the women that I've ever been with have been one-night stands or just some weekenders.

I got involved with a motorcycle gang in my early twenties, because I thought that was another step into Aussie manhood, of proving yourself. Looking back at it now, what a sense of waste of my life and the damage that I've done to other people, even though, like, people have done other things to me. But I always pushed people away, because of having the fear of being hurt, not trusting anybody, relying on my own instincts.

Making friends with a man in a Christian motorcycle club had been instrumental in helping Rod to overcome his past. He had been able to talk about himself for the first time in a safe environment. Rod described how his own thinking had gradually changed and how the 'real me' had emerged when he had started to write about his feelings and the events of his childhood.

And I eventually shared with a couple of people a little bit of information of what had happened to me as a kid, of being abused, because I knew I could trust these people. It was actually a Christian friend of mine that was involved in a Christian motorcycle club. Now I don't have to sort of hide behind a façade. Like I always felt comfortable with all the bikie gear on, hiding behind that, knowing people would feel threatened and would leave you alone. But, really, it was me isolating myself away from society. It was like being in solitary confinement, in prison in that regard through my own doing.

I tried to find other ways of dealing with the trauma that was locked inside of me, and I found that the best way to deal with it was to write. I wouldn't say that I was illiterate but I started going to college, picking up with reading, writing, spelling. And the teachers there highlighted little things to me and said, 'You seem to have a bit of a flair for writing.' And from there on, being able to express in words what was in here [points to heart] and in here [points to head] in poetry, it slowly started to come out. Putting pen to paper was a way of expressing those feelings that I had locked away for so long.

Rod used his appearance as a biker to keep both men and women at a distance. He worried that, if he had a girlfriend, she might turn out to be like his aunt. He still experienced feelings of rage bubbling up inside him, especially when he had been drinking. He knew how easy it would be for him to hurt, or even kill, a woman if he lost control or allowed his rage to take over. As a result he had made a decision that it was safer for everyone if he only had very short relationships, or one-night stands, with women. I was saddened by this choice.

> I was frightened that if I had a woman and I drank, all that explosive energy would come out and that I would beat the crap out of her, or maybe even kill her. So I made a decision that I would not take that step for fear of doing damage to the partner. So that's why all my sexual relationships with women were always one-night stands. And I realise how much I've missed out on. But I don't have the patience for kids. I know my own tolerance I suppose. I just don't have the tolerance and the patience for kids. I could do damage.

The gender socialisation of Australian men like Rod

As part of the gender socialisation process in Australia, young boys like Rod are taught not to express their emotions, but this emotional inexpressiveness has many negative consequences for them.[8] Emotions associated with vulnerability, such as fear or sadness, are particularly taboo. These unacceptable emotions are often replaced with anger, which is seen as an acceptable male emotion.[9] As a result, young boys who have experienced childhood sexual abuse often have difficulty coming to terms with their experiences. 'In our society, masculinity is organised as "not feminine", or, more bluntly, "not effeminate".'[10] Masculinity is constructed through a boy's separation from his mother. This involves rejecting his feminine aspects, in order to develop a masculine identity. Men are socialised, to varying degrees, not to show feminine traits such as weakness or vulnerability. In the same way, young boys receive strong societal messages that same-sex attraction and homosexual experience must remain hidden.[11]

'The typical Australian male, whether we talk about the bushman, the battler, the larrikin, or the suburban ocker, understands masculinity as machismo and thinks that "being masculine" means being tough, forceful and aggressively defensive.'[12] Young boys learn to be disconnected from others, to see sex as a goal in its own right, and some men like Rod develop serious problems with non-relational sex.[13] It seems to me that Rod paid a high price for his childhood sexual experience. He decided not to enter into intimate relationships with women and he suffered from the typical mental health problems experienced by men following sexual abuse, including risk-taking behaviour, aggression, somatic problems, and alcohol or drug abuse.[14] Will's story also reflects some of these difficulties.

Will's story – 'never considered myself a victim'

Will was a social worker in his late sixties. He was brought up by foster parents whom he believed were his biological parents. He was looked after mainly by his foster father's mother. His first sexual experience was at junior school. Later on his foster father put him into a boys' home and he tried to run away many times. On two of these occasions he was sexually abused by men that he met while on the run. At the time he blamed himself and told no one.

Will learned how to fight and to defend himself at the boys' homes. He was tall and strong and used his aggression and authority to prevent younger boys from being raped by older boys. He described much of the sexual activity within the home as experimentation, fuelled by curiosity and boredom. He believed that when the boys left the home they walked away from that as well.

> My first experience of abuse was my first day at school. The older boys took the infant boys and fooled around with them. There was lowering of pants, and some penetration by these boys. And it was all a mystery. The chap who I thought was my father was overseas, and the lady I thought was my mother wasn't about very much. I was in the care of the grandmother who didn't particularly like me. She used to call me a 'shithouse rat just like my mother' actually. And she wasn't a person I'd talk to about anything, because I was always to blame no matter what happened. So you kept that sort of thing to yourself. That only happened the once; they never touched me again. And there was no physical violence.
>
> They put me in a boys' home, and I absconded from there several times, and it was during two occasions that I was picked up by a bloke, taken home, basically raped, although I didn't think it at the time. I thought I was to blame, because I'd run away and therefore I'd put myself in that situation. He took me home. His mother was there and she proudly told me who he was. He had a fairly high position in the courts. And during the night he's in bed with me, and I woke up to find him doing things to me. Once again there was a lot of confusion, mainly because his mother seemed to be involved. I never told anyone at the home. Every time I went back I got a belting, and they were pretty savage beltings. The superintendent, a minister, used to lose his cool occasionally and really get stuck into you.
>
> I absconded again and this bloke met me in a park. I was looking for somewhere to sleep. We met and we talked and I told him some story but he sussed it out, and so it was virtually, 'If you don't cooperate . . .' But it was oral sex on me, which I wasn't too keen on. Then he said it's your turn, and I wouldn't. He called me all sorts of things, and a couple of nights later the police turned up.

Will seemed to enjoy talking about his childhood spent in various boys' homes. He spoke almost affectionately about the other boys and the various fights he had been involved in. He was obviously a bright child and tried to protect the younger boys in whatever way he could.

> There were attempts in the home, but by the time that I got there I was starting to get a bit street-wise. Boys tried it on, but by that time I'd decided that I'd handle anybody that tried it on. I'm about 13 or 14 by this stage, and I've always been tall and fairly fit. There were a few kids who were starting to rape little blokes. Well, we sorted them out. They thought they were easy meat. Well, they weren't.
>
> The other boys were egging me on to have a go at this boy, and I knew I could beat him. But suddenly I realised that this was all entertainment. And so I decided there and then I wouldn't. I came to a conclusion that you don't give anything any more power or any more victory over you than it deserves. I've maintained that with those characters too that abused me, the children and the two blokes. I just won't let it be an influence on me, never have.

Will strongly disliked the intense media coverage and the people in the media who focused on this issue. He saw them as parasites building their careers on the misfortune of others. He believed that the way in which they treated the victim was another form of violation and re-victimisation. He remained defiant and determined not to be defined by his childhood sexual experiences.

> There was a degree of shame because I didn't feel shame. When you've got these parasites that build up careers on 'these poor broken people whose lives are ruined', they convey a message that you should feel something terrible because this has happened to you. That's their message: you're ruined. Stuff them. But you think, 'Well, maybe they're right. Maybe there is something wrong with me, in that I don't get all uptight and angry about it.'
>
> I feel for women who are raped. It's bad enough that they are assaulted and they're abused, but for society to be saying they're been dirtied, I reckon that's garbage. And it's bad enough in our culture. In other cultures, they kill the women that have been raped. It's not that we're any more civilised, it's only various degrees removed from the patriarchal garbage. So I don't carry a lot of luggage about it. Anybody wants to know, I'll talk about it because I don't think I've done anything wrong.

Will strongly believed that anyone who had been maltreated in childhood needed to take responsibility for their own behaviour, because they knew the impact of such experiences on others. He was adamant that his life had not been ruined by his experiences.

> I had counselling for about a year. But the abandonment issues were the big thing, by the people I thought were carers. Not those blokes. I talked about it,

couldn't care less about it, but it wasn't a big issue. I think you carry emotional scars. I've never considered myself a victim, never. I think that takes away your humanity, if you're considered a victim. No matter what happens to you, you know whether something's right or wrong. And if you've been battered and bruised yourself, and if you've been betrayed, you know what it is to betray. And then you turn around and betray someone else. Don't tell me that you're not responsible, because you know better than people who've never been betrayed.

Will described himself as a lost soul, on a downward spiral, and in and out of jail. He became involved with a church through becoming suicidal. Things were going well for him briefly, until he stole from the church. He had a conversion experience and decided to return to the church. Instead of being met with anger and rejection, he was welcomed back with open arms. The impact of this on Will was profound and he decided to pay back all the money he had stolen. This eventually led his life in a new direction of helping others.

> Later on I'd been in and out of jail and I deserved to be. I was stealing from people. I was thinking suicidal things, and rang Lifeline. I got involved with the church and was going great guns until I shot through with their money. Then I had an hour with this psychiatrist. He talked me into going back to this church, and they were what the Gospel talks about. When I walked in, you would have thought they had won Lotto. Their faces lit up, and I'd knocked off a lot of money from them, and they couldn't have been more accepting and more loving. And that's when I had this conversion experience. And I worked a double shift for a year, and got enough money to pay back money I'd stolen.

Will's refusal to be labelled as a 'victim'
Will refused to accept the idea that his life had been ruined by the events of his childhood. He refused to accept that he was a victim or that he should be seen as an object of pity in any way. This may partly be because of the way in which masculine identity is constructed. Young boys like Will know that they are not supposed to be dependent, weak, vulnerable or passive. As a result, they suppress their feelings of emotional vulnerability and demonstrate more acceptable, traditionally masculine behaviour such as behaving aggressively and demonstrating anger rather than sadness. It is often difficult for young boys and men to seek help and to be emotionally vulnerable.[15] Will believed that the physical abuse, neglect and abandonment that he experienced had more impact on his life than the childhood sexual abuse. But, above all, he believed that it was necessary to get on with life, rather than blame your past for your present.

NARRATIVE OF REMAINING DEFIANT

This was a feisty group of people who disliked being categorised or stigmatised by others. They refused to be labelled or pigeonholed as victims, or as survivors. They told a *narrative of remaining defiant*. They had all grown up in abusive environments and experienced physical, emotional and sexual abuse from a young age. They recognised the impact that these events had on them as children and as adults. However, they refused to be defined by these events or to have their identities linked to them. They wanted to be viewed as people in their own right. Two out of five had arrived at this conclusion with little or no help from professionals.

Everyone in this group had learned to push away thoughts about their childhood sexual experiences. They didn't see any benefit to dwelling on such experiences, and refused to allow them to dominate their lives. Instead they longed to be normal and to live normal lives. They chose not to tell anyone as children, apart from Belinda whose story was uncovered by her stepmother. Perhaps their desire to be seen as 'normal' influenced their decision not to tell. Rod was driven by his fear of being thought to be homosexual. He wanted to avoid this shame at all cost and therefore didn't want family members or anyone else to know what had happened to him.

These men and women knew that their childhood sexual experiences had a profound impact on them throughout their lives. This made it all the more remarkable that they had found such strength and refused to be seen as victims or to be defined by their childhood experiences. They knew that they had behaved aggressively or violently as young adults in response to their experiences. During their late adolescence they all, except for Belinda, became aggressive and deliberately tried to hurt people. They were not necessarily aware of their motives at the time but, looking back, they could recognise their use of alcohol and drugs as a self-destructive pattern and their aggressive behaviour as a form of revenge.

At certain times during their lives they had either felt suicidal or had reverted to excessive use of drugs or alcohol. Many of them experienced physical or sexual problems, and had been involved in non-committed sex. All had experienced difficulties with trusting people and with forging intimate relationships with others.

These men and women were on paths towards spiritual growth and healing, and to working in the helping professions. This was a common theme that linked them in that all of them found comfort and acceptance within a faith community of some kind. The changes in Rod were more subtle and less dramatic. Although their stories had a spiritual quality to them, they were told in an earthy manner. These were down-to-earth men and women who longed to be seen as normal, rather than as somehow damaged.

In the next chapter I will look at the issue of telling or not telling across all

22 men and women interviewed, and will illuminate some interesting gender differences in disclosure and non-disclosure.

SUMMARY

Key points

- These five men and women were *remaining defiant* and refusing to be defined by their childhood sexual experiences.
- They longed to be seen as normal, rather than as damaged goods or as victims of child sexual abuse, as portrayed in the media.
- They knew that they had been severely affected by what had happened to them and had worked hard at overcoming the impact that being maltreated as children had on their lives.
- However, they believed that they were greater than the sum of their childhood experiences and didn't want to have their identities linked solely to these experiences.
- They believed that being seen as either a victim or a survivor of child sexual abuse was stigmatising.
- They spoke, in a down-to-earth manner, of their spiritual growth and of transcending their childhood experiences.

CHAPTER 9

Kids and adults that don't tell

INTRODUCTION

> **Chapter aims**
> - Examine the issue of disclosure and non-disclosure of childhood sexual experiences.
> - Describe the main inhibitors to disclosure among children.
> - Identify gender differences in terms of disclosure.
> - Illustrate the negative consequences of trying to tell an adult, as children.
> - Outline the ways in which, as adults, some people choose to make purposeful disclosures whereas others choose to make selective disclosures.
> - Describe the lifelong process of disclosure.

In this chapter, the issue of disclosure and non-disclosure is examined. Seventeen out of 22 of these men and women told no one what was happening to them as children, and many kept their childhood sexual experiences to themselves well into adulthood. By definition, they had all told someone by the time the research was conducted, although for one man I was the first person that he had told in his life and several others had only told their intimate partners before. Making a disclosure seemed to be a difficult thing to achieve. The main inhibitors to telling as a child were described as fear, shame and self-blame. Fear was more commonly described as an inhibiting factor by women, and shame was more commonly described by men.

Five people did try to tell someone about what was happening to them as children. Unfortunately for them, their disclosures did not have the desired effect and did not significantly improve their situations. Three of these went on to report their victimisers to the police as adults and, as a result, two men went to jail for the crimes described in this book. The other victimisers, both men and women, were never charged for their crimes. Sadly, this is not atypical. In this chapter the cost of telling and not telling will be explored.

FEAR AS A INHIBITOR TO DISCLOSURE, ESPECIALLY FOR GIRLS

People often chose not to tell anyone as children because they were too afraid to do so. This was particularly true of the women, although some men were also willing to admit to being frightened as children. Similarly, shame was more commonly cited as a reason for not telling by men, although some women also admitted to feelings of shame about their childhood sexual experiences. These gender differences may be largely due to gender socialisation.[1]

Growing fear, threats and manipulation

Many of these children had good reason to be fearful, since they were growing up with violent, alcoholic fathers or stepfathers and mothers who, for whatever, reason, were unable to protect them. They knew that their victimisers were capable of violence and that they would be hurt physically if they resisted. Even though some of them were initially treated gently, the threat of violence tended to increase over time as they themselves started to fight against what was happening to them. They were often manipulated by fear of the consequences for others, which prevented them from telling anyone. Most believed that if they weren't being assaulted then their siblings would be hurt instead of them. It is likely that this belief was planted by their victimisers, and that there was more than a grain of truth in it anyway.

Karen described how the fear built up over the years. Initially, her father told her what they were doing together was a secret but, as she got older, he threatened her with violence if she told her mother anything. For many years his strategy worked and Karen kept quiet. Jane remained fearful of her father well into adulthood. She moved house every few months because 'the thought of him coming after me is still in my mind'.

Tina was afraid to tell anyone what was happening to her as a child. Initially, she had loved the attention that she received from her aunt's boyfriend, because her father had died when she was a baby. As time went by it stopped being fun but, by then, she believed that she would get into a lot of trouble if she told anyone. She was frightened that her aunt would be angry with her and blame her for what had happened.

Belinda was cleverly manipulated by her stepfather. He convinced her that she was a home-wrecker and had caused the breakdown of her parents' marriage. He also kept the stepsisters apart by telling them how different they were. Belinda didn't want to break up her second family and she was very 'scared of rocking the family boat'. She was also concerned for her stepsister because 'all I ever wanted was a dad, and so I didn't want her to not have that'.

Fear of not being believed or being punished

Many of these children were afraid of the possible consequences if they told anyone what was happening to them. They often thought that they wouldn't be believed and that they would be accused of lying. They thought that the adult's word would be accepted and not theirs. They also believed that they would be punished for making such a statement. This was probably a reasonable assessment in many cases, since the few children who did try to tell were not believed, were punished and were made to continue to live with their victimisers.

For example, Bert believed that in his family 'it was actually safer to keep the secret than it was to be open about it'. Similarly, Peter decided that his mother would not believe that he had been sexually abused by a male cousin on his mother's side of the family. 'I don't think she would have wanted to believe that could happen, from within her own family.' He thought that she would gloss over the incident and say, 'Let's forget about it and move on.' This coincided with what he chose to do himself.

Bert believed that, for him, the consequences of telling would be worse than the consequences of not telling, in that he would probably be punished, and 'if I tell someone, it's going to be way, way worse'. Bert believed that if he tried to discuss it he would get into trouble for doing so. He went on to argue that, as a child, he thought that his parents didn't know anything about sex or homosexuality anyway.

Diana had several reasons for not telling anyone about her experiences. She knew that you were not supposed to tell outsiders and bring shame to bear on the good name of the family. When Diana was four, a man on the bus 'put his hand in my pants'. Afterwards her parents had decided to do nothing and Diana had been told by her mother not to tell anyone, thereby setting the scene for Diana to keep the rapes a secret later on.

Fear of consequences for others

As adults, these men and women also discussed their fears for other people in their families. These may have been post-rationalisations or they may have intuitively known, even as children, that the consequences of telling could be disastrous for others in some way. Their main fears were that their parents would act in a violent manner towards the victimiser, or that their siblings would end up being sexually abused instead of them. There is certainly some evidence that the second of these fears was well founded.

Both Diana and Peter felt protective towards their parents. As children they believed that their fathers would murder their victimisers if they ever found out what had happened. As Diana said, 'My father would be in jail for murder, if he found out about this.' Peter was as frightened for himself as for what his father might do to him and his cousin. He described himself as 'petrified about, not only what Dad would dish out to the other family, but what he'd dish out to me'.

Several people described feeling afraid for their siblings. As many as 10 of them found out, as adults, that their siblings had also been sexually abused, which suggests that their concerns were entirely justified. For example, Heather decided when she was young not to tell anyone in order to protect her younger siblings. She even chose to sleep on the bottom bunk, believing that if she was being sexually abused this would protect them from the same fate. This pattern of trying to protect siblings was very common.

SHAME AS AN INHIBITOR TO DISCLOSURE, ESPECIALLY FOR BOYS

Many of the men described their homophobic responses to their childhood sexual experiences. These took several forms: fear that they would be labelled by others as homosexual if their experiences were known publicly; that they were chosen by their victimisers because of their own hidden homosexuality; or that they themselves would become homosexual as a result of their homosexual experiences. In other words they were concerned about the stigma of being labelled homosexual or that their homosexuality was either the cause or would be the unwanted effect of their childhood experiences. Whether these feelings of shame were encouraged by the victimiser or stemmed from societal beliefs about homosexuality is hard to determine.

For the three out of nine men who had sexual experiences with women during childhood, feelings of shame and confusion were also evident since their experiences contradicted gender expectations.

Shame about being labelled as gay

Peter was worried that people would find out what had happened to him and label him as gay. He decided that he would 'never ever mention it to them [his close male friends], never ever, and I wouldn't' in case they thought he was homosexual. As Rod became an adolescent he began to realise the stigma attached to being seen as homosexual and he became even more determined that no one would find out about what had happened to him. He started drinking partly to overcome his 'sense of extreme rage and hatred towards people like that'. Colin also feared being seen as gay as a result of his experiences with his brother.

Shame about hidden homosexuality

Some men were concerned that they might have been selected by their victimisers because they were believed to be homosexual. For example, Leo thought that he 'must have had victim written all over my face'. Jim questioned why he had been singled out by his teacher for physical punishment and sexual abuse. 'I'm sure he wasn't doing it to anyone else, what he was doing to me. Why he had me isolated I don't know?' Some of his intense sense of shame was attached to this.

On the other hand Bert, who was bisexual, did not believe that his early homosexual experiences had changed his sexual orientation in any way. He believed that his sexuality predated these experiences.

Shame about becoming homosexual

The intensity of the shame experienced by some of the men was great. For example, Rod described how ashamed he felt when he realised the homosexual nature of his experiences. This was intensified by the fear that it could actually make him become homosexual. As previously described, Rod coped with this fear by becoming violently homophobic. It is significant that he uses the expression 'taking away my manhood', which suggests that he felt emasculated by what happened.

Confusion about heterosexual experiences for boys

When the men described heterosexual experiences with older women in childhood, they expressed a great deal of confusion about these experiences. For example, Angelo believed that his male friends would have laughed at him or seen him as lucky if he had told them that he had had childhood sexual experiences with women. For Norm and Leo, the experiences were very different in nature because they involved their mothers. They felt a great deal of shame and confusion about what had happened and to what extent they were culpable themselves. They felt extreme anger towards their mothers. It was very difficult for them to talk about their experiences, which they knew to be taboo, even in today's society.

SELF-BLAME AS AN INHIBITOR TO DISCLOSURE

Self-blame was a powerful reason for not telling anyone about childhood sexual experiences. Several blamed themselves and took on the responsibility for what had happened to them as children. Even as adults, many of them continued to blame themselves for not being able to prevent the abuse or stop it from happening. This is a terrible testimony to the ability of their victimisers to manipulate these children. It may also be a reflection of the societal view that victims of sexual assault somehow ask for it. It seems so sad and so incredibly unfair that a child should take on the blame for the adult's abusive actions. It also plays into the hands of victimisers, who are able to manipulate the situation to their own advantage.

Victoria felt that she was to blame for not being able to stand up to her mother and stepfather as an adolescent. She believed that by the age of 16 she should have been able to extricate herself from the situation somehow. She felt ashamed that she had been unable to do so, and this had been another reason not to tell anyone about what had happened. Her shame increased in adolescence and adulthood, as she began to understand more of what had happened.

Diana wanted to protect her mother from feeling guilty that she had failed to protect Diana as a child. She thought that the knowledge of her rape would be devastating to her mother, with whom she remained close. Diana preferred to accept the blame for what happened and to believe that she was responsible for being raped because she went to a particular part of town, despite her mother's warning not to go there.

For many years Jewels felt dirty, ashamed and responsible for what had happened to her. As an adult she was no longer willing to remain silent about her experiences but she had to overcome her feelings of guilt in order to speak up. This was true for other men and women, too, who needed to get to a position of believing that they were not responsible before they could speak up about the crime that had been perpetrated against them.

NEGATIVE CONSEQUENCES OF TELLING AS A CHILD

Non-disclosure was far more common than disclosure in childhood. Seventeen people did not tell anyone as a child about their sexual experiences with adults. However, four of them did describe behaving in ways that they now wished had been recognised as expressions of their distress. For example, Jane and her twin had gone to school covered in bruises which the teachers had ignored. As an adult, Jane found it hard to understand why the neighbours had never complained or stepped in to help given that 'the violence that we had to endure, there were many times that we would be screaming our heads off'. Diana described how she carried a knife as a young woman and attacked men. Norm and Rod both acted violently as young men, hoping that someone would realise their situation.

Five people, four women and one man, had tried to tell as children that they were being sexually abused but none of them believed that telling had helped them or improved their situation in any significant way. In fact, their experiences of trying to tell were traumatic in themselves. Those who tried to tell as children suffered many different negative consequences as a result of their attempts at disclosure. Three were not believed and two were asked to choose whether or not the victimiser should stay in the home or not. As a result nothing changed for the better as a result of telling an adult. This may have fuelled their feelings of anger and increased the likelihood of them reporting their victimiser to the police as adults.

Not being believed

Hope, Leo, Tina and Karen all told their mothers what was happening to them. As a very young child Hope told her mother that her vagina was sore and bleeding and her mother did nothing about it. She blamed Hope for the situation, telling her that she was masturbating too much. As an adult Hope felt some sympathy for her mother, whom she believed had been 'a victim of serial child rape herself' and was 'so traumatised and hadn't dealt with it'. But her tone was angry when she described how her mother had ignored her needs and placed the blame on her as a child.

Leo and Tina both had mothers who ignored their disclosures. They were simply not believed. Tina felt responsible for being sexually abused by her aunt's boyfriend. At the age of nine, she found out that he was doing the same thing to a cousin. The girls decided to tell their uncle, as a result of which the sexual abuse stopped for her cousin, but not for Tina. It was to continue until she was 16 years old. Tina repeatedly told other family members, but they all chose to do nothing about the situation. Paradoxically, this lack of action may have helped Tina to decide to make a report to the police as an adult.

Being asked to choose and nothing changing

When people disclosed what was happening to them as children, their families did not respond appropriately or in a supportive manner. Their situations didn't improve and, as a result, some of them felt betrayed and angry. It is possible that this anger helped them to disclose what had happened to them later as adults. Some of their anger was focused on their victimisers, but they also felt angry with their mothers for failing to listen to them, or take responsibility and protect them.

When Karen told her mother, she was asked to choose whether or not she wanted her father to stay or to leave. Karen felt unable to ask for him to leave, because she was afraid that her mother would hate her for splitting up the family. As a result she had to continue to live with her father. Later in life she discovered that he had sexually abused all of his five children, including his son. Belinda was also asked to choose the fate of her stepfather. Not surprisingly, she made the same decision with similar consequences. She had to continue to live in the same household as her victimiser.

TELLING AS AN ADULT

There is a difference between telling the police or the family involved and telling someone else like an intimate partner, friend or therapist. I have used the term *purposeful disclosure* to describe telling the police or the family involved, and the term *selective disclosure* to describe telling someone who was not involved or was unlikely to take any action as a result of knowing. There were 10 people who made *purposeful disclosures* as adults, most of whom were women. There were 12 people, including most of the men, who made *selective disclosures* as adults. In some ways the *selective disclosures* continued to protect their victimisers from the consequences of the abuse, and may partly have been self-protective measures.

PURPOSEFUL DISCLOSURE, ESPECIALLY BY WOMEN

Of the five people who tried to tell someone in childhood, all but one went on to make purposeful disclosures as adults. An additional six other women also made purposeful disclosures in adulthood. Of these 10 people, nine were women. Five made full reports to the police and five confronted their families. These disclosures had considerable consequences for those involved in terms of disruption to their family relationships. The lack of family support following disclosure was often seen as an act of betrayal.

Telling the police

Jane felt obliged to report her father to the police when she realised that he was sexually abusing his 12-year-old stepdaughter. She wanted to prevent him from sexually assaulting other children. She felt a sense of relief as if a 'huge burden lifted off my shoulders' when she stood up to her father in this way. The police were unable to prosecute him over Jane's abuse, but he was arrested for abusing his stepdaughter and was sent to jail. Jane was cynical and did not believe that his jail sentence had any real effect on him at all.

Hope and Colin also made reports to the police but no prosecutions had been made to date on their behalf. Colin was unemployed and had decided to seek compensation through the courts. Although he had talked to the police, he was still reluctant to talk to his children and other family members about what happened.

Karen decided to report her father to the police when she was 32, in response to an advertising campaign by police. This campaign implied that if you failed to report a victimiser you were as guilty as they were. She felt a burden lift from her shoulders and was excited that something was finally going to be done to make her father take responsibility for his actions. Going to court, Karen felt frightened. She knew that this was an automatic response, but she had to constantly reassure herself by saying that she was in the right, and that her father was in the wrong.

Karen had hoped that her mother would support her and her siblings during the trial. She was devastated by what she saw as a betrayal when her mother chose to sit beside Karen's father in court and to support him throughout. Her mother also told the court 'we were compulsive liars when we were younger'. From that point onwards in her story Karen called her mother by her first name rather than calling her 'Mum'. It was as if she no longer considered her to be her mother, after betraying her children during the trial. Her father was found guilty, went to jail and died there.

There was an element of *selective disclosure* even within Karen's story of *purposeful disclosure*. Karen and her sisters decided to prosecute their father without revealing that their brother had also been sexually abused. Although Karen did not agree with her brother's decision to hide his sexual abuse, she and her siblings understood his desire not to be publicly labelled as a victim. She accepted that this might have caused him problems in his work environment.

Tina explained that it took a long time before she decided to go to the police as an adult because she was 'just so fragile'. Again 'probably the family's betrayal is actually more painful' to bear than the actual assaults by her aunt's boyfriend. Tina was happy that the police had taken her statement seriously, but she was also relieved that she did not have to go to court, because her victimiser was too elderly by that time for the police to charge him.

For Belinda, the anger and frustration that she felt about her situation had grown over the years. Recently, her mother had briefly separated from her stepfather and during that time Belinda felt safe enough to tell her more of what had happened in her childhood. When her mother decided to go back to live with him, Belinda found this even more difficult to deal with. It seemed like a betrayal and left her feeling even angrier.

Lack of family support following disclosure seen as betrayal

Most people who told their families as adults received little or no support from them. Some, like Heather, felt further betrayed by her mother when the story of the sexual abuse by her father emerged. Heather's mother denied that incest had ever taken place. She rejected Heather and accused her of fabricating the whole story. When Heather separated from her husband and was setting up house with a female partner, her mother sided with Heather's husband and took out a court order to prevent Heather from gaining custody of the children. Having been so close to her mother as a young child and having believed that she had protected her mother from domestic violence at the hands of her violent father, Heather was devastated by what she saw as a betrayal by her mother.

Victoria and her sister Tess did not need to tell their mother about their sexual abuse at the hands of their stepfather because she had condoned his behaviour. This was very confusing to both girls who were angrier with their mother than their stepfather.

The only person who was supported by her mother following a disclosure made in adulthood was Sylvia. After an initial period where she found it hard to accept what her daughter was telling her, her mother decided to support her recovery process and began to remember events that corroborated her story.

SELECTIVE DISCLOSURE, ESPECIALLY BY MEN

It wasn't easy for some people to make disclosures, even as adults. As a result 12 people made only *selective disclosures*. The men seemed to find it particularly difficult, perhaps because many of the inhibitors to disclosure still existed for them. For some of the women, their fear had diminished over the years and been replaced by anger, whereas for some of the men their feelings of shame remained. For some people it had become a habit not to talk about it, whereas others still wanted to protect their families from knowing what had happened to them. Some had started to feel guilty about not telling the police and preventing future child sexual abuse.

Learned not to talk about it

Norm described how he had quickly learned not to talk about his early sexual experiences because his peers knew so much less than he did. He acknowledged that he still didn't find his experiences comfortable to talk about and that he was saying as little as possible about actual events during the interview.

Angelo had only recently started to think about the possible impact that his experiences might have had on him. He had been brought up in a traditional Catholic family and still found the idea of telling his Italian parents unimaginable, since sex and sexuality were taboo topics. Angelo also believed that his male friends would dismiss his sexual experiences with women as harmless, or even view him as fortunate for having had them.

As previously described, Diana never wanted her mother to know that she had been raped. Peter's reason for choosing not to tell his parents as an adult was also a desire not to upset them in their old age. This was also reflected by Jewels. Leo had only started to recover memories of abuse by his mother after her death.

Recently feeling guilty about not telling police

Peter had been reviewing his decision in recent years and was concerned that he might have caused other children to be hurt by protecting his family. He still wanted to protect his elderly parents, but he also felt distraught at the thought that he should have done more. He became tearful in the interview when discussing this. He had begun to feel under increasing pressure to report what had happened to him many years ago. Peter described how 'it was so much in the media, and it brought it back into my mind again that maybe I had done the wrong thing in not reporting it'. He returned to this concern several times during the interview. He was also concerned that his cousin now lived near one of his relatives. He told himself that she was safe, but a seed of doubt had been planted in his mind.

In this chapter I have examined the issue of disclosure as a lifelong process that is challenging for many children. I have also suggested that disclosure may be easier for women than for men and that *purposeful disclosure* may be more common among women, whereas *selective disclosure* may be more common among men. These findings raise many issues for discussion.

In the next chapter, I discuss the five resilient narratives told by these men and women in greater detail. And in the following chapter, I look at the impact of the changing social discourse around child sexual abuse, the impact of the family context on narrative development, and gender similarities and differences in both disclosure and narrative development.

SUMMARY

Key points
- Non-disclosure was far more common than disclosure.
- Disclosure of childhood sexual experiences was a complex process. Most people chose not to tell anyone during childhood, and many only made selective disclosures as adults. Coming out about childhood sexual experiences was challenging, even for adults.
- The main factors inhibiting children from telling anyone were fear, shame and self-blame.
- Many children, especially girls, were afraid of being hurt or punished if they told anyone what was happening to them. They were also afraid of not being believed and of the possible consequences for other members of their families if they did tell.
- Many children, particularly boys, felt too ashamed of what was happening to them to tell an adult. They were ashamed that they might be labelled as homosexual by other people if they found out what had happened. Some were afraid that they had been chosen because of their own hidden homosexuality, or that they might become homosexual as a result of their experiences.
- There was a tendency for children and, in particular, for adolescents to blame themselves for what was happening to them. They often felt responsible for not stopping or preventing the abuse. This feeling often persisted well into adulthood.
- Some children showed signs of distress that were not picked up by the adults around them. Others tried to tell an adult, usually their mothers, but were not believed or were accused of lying. Their situations as children did not significantly improve as a result of telling and some were asked to choose what should happen to their victimiser.
- It is possible that trying to tell as a child, and not being believed, fuelled a desire to seek justice in adulthood and the decision to report the victimiser to

the police. *Purposeful disclosure* was more common among women but came at considerable personal cost, and the resultant betrayal by the family and the lack of family support was often seen as worse than the abuse itself.

- Most men, and a few women, made only *selective disclosures* about their childhood sexual experiences, even as adults. They continued to feel the need to protect themselves and their family members from the pain of knowing into adulthood.
- Some people were starting to feel guilty about not having told the police, in order to protect children from being hurt in the future.

CHAPTER 10

Drawing together the threads of resilience

INTRODUCTION

> **Chapter aims**
> - Describe the way in which people become the narratives that they tell.
> - Draw together the threads of resilience in the six narratives told by these men and women.
> - Identify the complexities in these six narratives:
>   — *narrative of normal sexual development*
>   — *narrative of a silence recently broken*
>   — *narrative of the need to remember and the need to forget*
>   — *narrative of protecting and helping others*
>   — *narrative of justice at any cost*
>   — *narrative of remaining defiant.*

This chapter draws together the interwoven threads of the various narratives told and examines the overall pattern, texture and colour of the tapestry created by the men and women interviewed. It seems to me that most of them managed to arrive at a point in their lives where the narratives that they told were of resilience and courage, in the face of often horrendous child maltreatment. This had not been an easy journey for many of them, given their family backgrounds, but they had achieved it nonetheless and created a colourful tapestry of their lives.

NARRATIVE CONSTRUCTION OF THE SELF

From a social constructionist perspective, people live within a culture and its stories and are influenced by and influence these narratives.[1] We construct narratives to explain to ourselves, and to others, the story of our lives. In a sense, we become the narratives that we tell about ourselves since we are relational beings, and we construct a sense of who we are through dialogue with others. I was interested in understanding the narratives told by people who had childhood sexual experiences with adults and found them to be *narratives of resilience*. By that I mean the narratives that people told me described how they had overcome their childhood adversity, in various ways, and had developed a positive sense of themselves in relation to, or despite, their childhood experiences.

Each man or woman told a narrative that, from a social constructionist perspective,[2] was a reconstruction of events within the context of the interview and did not necessarily represent what had actually happened in their life. The narrative reflected the current developmental perspective of that person. It was created within the context of the person's experiences within their own family, culture, social class, race and the context of the times. It was a narrative told to a specific person, in a specific context (i.e. the research interview), for a specific reason (e.g. the need to have the story heard or the desire to help others, etc.).

In some cases these narratives enabled these men and women to develop a social identity by identifying with members of already existing groups. For example, those telling *narratives of the need to remember and the need to forget* embraced the social identity of a victim and those telling *narratives of protecting and helping others* or *justice at any cost* were comfortable with the social aspects of the role of survivor of child sexual abuse. In contrast, those telling *narratives of remaining defiant* felt threatened by the desire of others to categorise them and refused to be stereotyped in this way.[3]

How do children develop positive self-esteem, a sense of mastery and agency in the world, an ability to keep themselves and others safe, and a capacity to trust and to be intimate with others?[4] These are some of the life challenges that are made more complicated and potentially problematic for children who have had childhood sexual experiences with adults. So how do most of these children develop into well-adjusted adults and competent and loving parents?

Although some of the men and women interviewed were still struggling with these difficulties (*narratives of the need to remember and the need to forget*), many appeared to have either passed through the eye of the storm (*narratives of protecting and helping others, justice at any cost*, or *defiance*) or managed to avoid the full force of the storm so far (*narratives of normal sexual development* or *a silence recently broken*). Most had managed to develop a self-narrative that helped them to feel good about themselves despite, or in some cases because of, their childhood sexual experiences. The process varied according to the six different narratives.

THE SIX NARRATIVES OF RESILIENCE

Men and women in this study told *narratives of resilience* in relation to their childhood sexual experiences. *Normal sexual development* was a controversial narrative that may fit for some adolescents who have sexual experiences where they believe that they are in control of the situation. *A silence recently broken* was a paradoxical narrative. The silence referred to wasn't the silence of the child, but the silence of the adult who has decided that she or he has not been affected by these experiences. The paradox lay in the fact that these adults did, nevertheless, come forward to be interviewed at a point in time when many of them were starting to question their own narrative.

The need to remember and the need to forget was a narrative told by people who felt little hope for the future and it had a 'stuck', less resilient quality as a narrative, similar to the victim discourse. These men and women were in the process of recovering memories or campaigning for other victims. *Protecting and helping others* and *justice at any cost* were survivor narratives told by those who, on the whole, felt that they had overcome their childhood adversity and had become protectors or helpers of others, or had helped to break the cycle of abuse for future generations. *Remaining defiant* was a resilient narrative of those who refused to be defined by their childhood experiences.

Although people were divided into six groups according to the main thrust of the narrative that they told at the time of the interview, it is important to remember that narratives can change over the course of time. For example, Sylvia, Tess and Leo told a victim narrative as a result of a process of realisation or of recovering memories. Others, like Jewels and Tina, described moving from a victim to a survivor narrative. Those telling *narratives of protecting and helping others or seeking justice at any cost* had been silenced when young, but they didn't tell a *narrative of a silence recently broken* because they didn't believe that they had been unaffected by their experiences. Each of these six narratives will be discussed in turn.

NARRATIVE OF NORMAL SEXUAL DEVELOPMENT

This narrative was told by one man and one woman who genuinely believed that they were unaffected by their early sexual experiences. They saw these experiences as part of their normal sexual development. They weren't concerned about the impact of these experiences and Greta believed that she had been in control of what had happened, to a large extent. They had a non-traumatic pathway into adulthood and were asymptomatic as children and as adults. Their childhood tapestries had been colourful and unblemished by these particular events.

Non-traumatic pathway into adulthood

For Greta and Bert their childhood sexual experiences had not been disturbing in any way. In fact they reported them as pleasurable. As Bert said, 'It was physically pleasurable and it was interesting, like it was "Wow." It was like a discovery.' Even though Bert felt some guilt because of the homosexual nature of his experiences, and thought that he would be punished if his parents knew what had happened, he didn't dwell on them and they didn't appear to impact negatively on his sense of who he was or his emerging sexual identity as a bisexual man.[5] Greta and Bert had both decided not to tell their families and had gone on to lead successful and fulfilling lives, including sexual experiences with people of both sexes. Bert knew that 'it's not an okay thing to say' in today's climate of opinion that he had been sexually abused as a child and that he was okay. Theirs appeared to be a non-traumatic journey into adulthood.

Asymptomatic children and adults

Greta and Bert described themselves as asymptomatic as children. They didn't believe that they suffered in any adverse way. They were similar to up to 40% of other children who experience child sexual abuse and remain asymptomatic. Like those telling a *narrative of a silence recently broken*, they may have been less affected as children because their experiences were less severe, they were more resilient, or they had a coping style that hid their distress.[6] It is thought that about 10% to 20% of these asymptomatic children will experience a deterioration in mental health at a later stage in their development and this has been termed the sleeper effect.[7] However, there is little research evidence about this phenomenon. Certainly, Greta and Bert didn't expect to develop problems in the future related to the past.

NARRATIVE OF A SILENCE RECENTLY BROKEN

The four men and women telling *narratives of a silence recently broken* were remarkable in that they started the interview by describing how their childhood sexual experiences hadn't impacted negatively on their lives. They hadn't experienced severe adjustment difficulties as adolescents or young adults. Instead they seemed able to accept what happened, decide not to dwell on it or talk about it, and move on with life. Until recently, remaining silent had been a pragmatic and non-problematic choice for them. Those men and women who told *narratives of a silence recently broken* either had no need to think about these events or had managed to put all thoughts of their childhood sexual experiences successfully out of their minds. For them, the tapestry of childhood had been reasonably colourful and bright, with only a few dark patches.

Victoria, Angelo, Jim and Peter admitted to some feelings of shame about their experiences, but they had chosen not to think about them at the time or to talk about them to anyone. They had moved through life reasonably success-fully, got married, had children and developed successful careers for themselves. Perhaps the only clue that they were having any difficulty at all was that they agreed to be interviewed. They had all reached a point in their lives where they were starting to question whether or not their childhood sexual experiences had affected them more than they had realised at the time, particularly within their intimate lives. In a sense they were starting to unravel the colourful tapestry of childhood and examine it more closely, to see whether or not there was a con-nection between the darker threads.

Taken at face value, this narrative suggests either that there can be non-traumatic pathways through childhood maltreatment or that people can be resilient in the face of adversity. One alternative interpretation is that they experienced a relational injury which they successfully hid from themselves and were in denial about the effect of their experiences. An alternative explanation is that the changing social debate conducted through the media about the issue of child sexual abuse caused them to question their own stories. Some of them had started to question whether they had, after all, been right to keep silent. They were also becoming increasingly concerned about their ability to sustain intimate connections with other people.

Lack of traumatic response – resilience or denial?

The way in which these men and women told their stories demonstrated a level of resilience in childhood, adolescence and adulthood. Despite having child-hood sexual experiences that could be described as traumatic, apart from Jim, they appeared to believe that they had not been traumatised in any way. Jim knew that he had been 'at the edge of being a complete zombie' following his experiences with a sadistic school teacher. However, others telling *narratives of a silence recently broken* had not experienced emotional difficulties, other than some feelings of shame, and had moved on successfully with their lives appar-ently without experiencing any form of post-traumatic response.

This lack of a traumatic response may partly be explained by the fact that, apart from Victoria, they all came from reasonably functional nuclear families and experienced relatively little physical or emotional abuse at home. Apart from Victoria, their childhood sexual experiences happened away from home and, apart from Peter, they began when they were over 10 years old. For Angelo and Jim, these experiences were not with family members and they ended when cir-cumstances changed. These factors may have made it slightly easier for them to develop a sense of agency in the world because they had not all experienced the traumagenic dynamics of sexual abuse identified by Finkelhor: traumatic sexu-alisation; betrayal; stigmatisation; and powerlessness or disempowerment.[8]

In many ways these narratives challenge the current conceptualisation of child sexual abuse as a series of traumatic events that leads to Complex PTSD or some other form of traumatic response.[9] Those telling *narratives of a silence recently broken* reported a non-traumatic pathway through their childhood sexual experiences even though some of them, like Victoria and Jim, had experienced events that amounted to a form of totalitarian control for a period of months or years.[10] They lived in relatively good family environments, used avoidant coping skills and refused to dwell on their experiences.

On the other hand, some of the men like Angelo, Jim and Peter had serious concerns about their ability to create and sustain intimate relationships in their adult lives. They may have experienced a relational injury and successfully hidden it from themselves for many years. This leads to a discussion as to whether or not their behaviour represents a form of resilience or of denial. Psychoanalytic theorists might argue that these men and women were in denial about the impact of their childhood sexual experiences and would need, at some time in the future, to re-experience these childhood events in order to achieve an abreaction[11] or in order to integrate the traumatic memories more fully. They might also theorise that they would be more vulnerable to becoming victimisers themselves, through identification with the aggressor[12] coupled with dissociation.[13]

A different way to look at their experiences is in terms of resilient behaviour. According to Rutter's definition of resilience as functioning well despite adversity,[14] resilient people would be those who experienced childhood difficulties but, due to a combination of personal, family and social protective factors, had not been badly affected by these experiences. They continue to function well despite their adversity. In this study, people telling *narratives of a silence recently broken* could be seen as resilient. These narratives have not been described previously in qualitative research studies into the issue of child sexual abuse. Most other studies have been based on clinical samples of survivors of child sexual abuse who, by definition, believed that they had been badly affected by their childhood maltreatment and were willing to be defined in relation to these experiences.

Questioning their own narrative

As adults, these men and women looked back at what they believed to be their choice to maintain silence and felt that it had been the right decision at the time and had helped them to move on with their lives. They had developed coping strategies and a positive self-narrative. However, publicity about paedophilia had made them start to question their own ideas in two ways. First, they had started to question whether or not they had, after all, done the right thing by keeping quiet about their experiences or whether this decision had allowed other children to be hurt. Second, they had begun to question whether they had been affected by their childhood sexual experiences, particularly in terms of their ability to sustain intimate relationships with other people.

In some ways, their own narrative had become socially unacceptable. For example, Peter still felt reluctant to talk publicly about his experiences with his older cousin. He also knew that it was not acceptable to say publicly, 'I've been through all this and it hasn't really affected me.' Nevertheless he believed 'what was done was wrong, perhaps enjoying it was wrong, but I've got on with my life'. However, he had started to ask himself difficult questions like: 'Has he abused somebody else? Has somebody been seriously hurt?' His recent separation from his wife and his extramarital affair had made him question his ability to have satisfying intimate relationships.

In a similar way, Angelo and Jim had also started to question their ability to sustain meaningful relationships with others. Having had so many extramarital affairs, Angelo had developed a sense of himself as successful with women. But recently he had become depressed and suicidal as a result of the sexual difficulties that he was experiencing within his second marriage. He was starting to think, 'Maybe I'm gay. No I can't be. I'm not gay,' and to attribute his problems to his childhood sexual experiences with women. He had also recognised that 'I can only have sex with women I despise'. Jim had started to worry that his B&D activities with women were not healthy and were a form of re-enactment of his childhood sexual experiences. He was also aware of his difficulty in maintaining long-term relationships with women and his tendency to move on from one woman to the next. 'I'm a bit of a bloody mongrel in that way . . . I don't ever want a bloody permanent relationship.'

This suggests that these men and women may have sustained a *relational injury* as a result of their childhood sexual experiences. These childhood wounds may have slowly festered, and prevented them from sustaining good relationships with those close to them. Like Jim, they may have found it difficult to connect with others and may have preferred to isolate themselves, even within a relationship. Like Angelo and Peter, they may have seen sex purely as a physical act without emotional intimacy. Like Victoria, they may have found it hard to trust anyone enough to talk to them about important issues. As a result, they have all experienced difficulties in relationships, possibly stemming from their childhood sexual experiences and the breaking of a significant bond of trust.

NARRATIVE OF THE NEED TO REMEMBER AND THE NEED TO FORGET

These narratives were told by five men and women who were still working through the impact of their childhood sexual experiences. They were trying to make sense of their experiences and were involved in an ongoing process of reconstructing a sense of self in relation to others. In many ways they were still suffering the effects of their childhood experiences. They identified themselves as victims of child sexual abuse and were struggling to come to terms with the profound impact of their childhood experiences.

Those telling *narratives of the need to remember and the need to forget* were still in the process of developing a sense of self and reconstructing their lives. The original tapestry of their childhood experiences was woven out of muted colours and, as a result of their recent realisations as adults, they were reworking it using a full range of threads. This process was both painful and arduous. This was particularly true for Sylvia, Tess and Leo who had only recently recovered memories or come to a realisation about the extent of their childhood abuse. They had used protective coping mechanisms during childhood such as active or purposeful forgetting or unconscious mechanisms such as dissociation or amnesia for memories of traumatic events. They had internalised messages from adults that they were to blame for what was happening to them which, in turn, led them to shut down emotionally at the time. Having recovered memories in adulthood, they were starting to view their lives differently. This left them feeling vulnerable and fragile, as victims often do.

Internalising shame and blame leading to fragmentation

Sylvia, Tess, Hope and Colin all adopted a mask, or an adapted sense of self, but in a less extreme manner than Leo. As children, they had internalised messages from their families that they were to blame for what was happening to them, and had buried their feelings and their memories. Sylvia described developing a confident exterior or 'outside shell. The inside was this mash, this huge deep dark hole.' Hope knew that she was not developing normally and tried to fit in with her peers by 'just going on raw instinct and intuition and what I thought was normal'. She explained that 'people who've had interrupted childhoods are good at putting on façades'.

As adults, these men and women had started to attribute some of their difficulties in adolescence and early adulthood to their childhood maltreatment, e.g. difficulties with self-esteem, an inability to trust others, and an inability to keep themselves safe and to prevent re-victimisation. This helped them to make sense of some of the chaos they had lived through earlier in their lives, by seeing it within the context of being victims of child sexual abuse. This also helped them to make sense of many experiences of re-victimisation in adolescence and early adulthood. They believed that others had also seen them as potential victims.

Leo had been diagnosed with dissociative identity disorder[15] and was attending therapy. He described the process of the fragmentation of his identity in great detail. He believed that he had been sexually abused by his mother and was told to 'put on a happy face, pretend that things are wonderful, don't show them your real pain inside'. He had come to believe that he had created 'alters'[16] [alter egos] as a way of coping. Living like a child protected him from feeling overwhelmed by 'massive shame' connected to some form of ritual abuse that he believed he had experienced.

Dissociative identity disorder is a controversial diagnosis, accepted by some clinicians and questioned by others.[17] Some researchers see 'alters' as metaphors for different emotional states whereas others see them as autonomous entities capable of independent action. Ross[18] argues that while some people have dissociative identity disorder that may be related to childhood maltreatment, others suffer from a form of dissociative identity disorder that may be related to poor therapy techniques. It can be very difficult for a clinician to determine whether or not the person is confused, lying, misinterpreting memories or is delusional. Some clinicians worry that such a diagnosis can lead to a worsening of symptoms, a breakdown in relationships and a tangled web of fantasies and memories.[19] However, the diagnosis often makes sense to the individual who is experiencing a sense of fragmentation.

Experiencing child sexual abuse can disrupt 'the social process through which identity is constructed'.[20] This disruption can lead to a great deal of confusion on the part of the child. Many children who have been sexually abused need to preserve their attachment bonds with their main caregivers, in order to survive. If these caregivers are also sexually abusive towards them, children sometimes adopt a 'contaminated, stigmatized identity' and sees themselves as evil in order to preserve their positive view of the victimiser.[21] This sense of contamination was most evident for Leo, who described how one of his alters 'still believes he was a very, very bad person' who had done something that was unforgivable.

As adolescents and young adults, these men and women had difficulty maintaining relationships. Some like Leo and Colin became involved with drug and alcohol use, which complicated their lives even further. Sylvia described how, in relationships with men, she had to struggle 'just to have a little corner of myself'. Colin believed that his experiences had arrested his emotional development and he was still angry and spent 'a lot of time punching doors and walls'. However, both he and Hope had found a purpose in their lives by becoming campaigners against child victimisation.

Strength through remembering and telling

Hope and Leo had tried to tell their mothers what was happening to them as children, but the others had all felt unable to tell anyone. However, they seemed to have benefited in different ways from telling their stories as adults. Sylvia, Tess and Leo had gained a better understanding of their previously chaotic lives, and Hope and Colin had gained a sense of agency and control. Sylvia, Leo and Colin still felt intense anger. To date, they had been unable to move out of this vortex of strong emotions or to develop a strong sense of themselves beyond being victims.

People experiencing child sexual abuse, particularly if it has been accompanied by violence from a young age, often have an extremely fragmented or distorted sense of themselves. There was a sense in which these men and women were still caught up in the abuse, and either had a very fragile sense of who they were as individuals or held on to a sense of themselves as victims, and continued to suffer as a result of their childhood injuries.

It is hard to determine why some people, like Jewels, 'really cling to that role' and believe 'I'm safer being a victim' whereas others who have had similar experiences manage to move from victim to survivor and beyond.[22] It is possible that this is part of a developmental process and that, given time, they will be able to redesign the tapestry of childhood into a pattern that incorporates a symbol of hope for the future that seems to be missing from the current design.

NARRATIVE OF PROTECTING AND HELPING OTHERS

Three women who had childhood sexual experiences within the family told a survivor *narrative of protecting and helping others*. They had overcome feelings of self-blame and had developed a relational sense of self out of their childhood experiences. These narratives were similar to the survivor narrative that is common in the literature and link the person's identity to their childhood experiences.

Overcoming self-blame and manipulation

Those telling *narratives of protecting and helping others* were all women who had incestuous experiences of one kind or another. All except Tina had grown up in abusive families and had experienced physical, emotional and sexual abuse as children from a very young age. Even though their childhood tapestry was thin and threadbare, they had reworked it to incorporate symbols of safety, protection and healing. They intended to provide a far better tapestry for their own children as they had the strong desire to protect and help others.

Constructing a strong self-narrative in a childhood that is characterised by maltreatment is a difficult task. Most believed that they were responsible for what was happening to them as children and blamed themselves, which has been shown to be more common among female survivors.[23] As adults, they had gradually come to the realisation that 'I'm not ashamed of it any more and I don't think it was my fault.'

Seeing self as protecting and helping others

Given that these women grew up in abusive families, they were not afforded sufficient protection by other family members including their mothers. Many went on to develop a relational sense of themselves as protectors of others and this was an important part of their belief system. Heather tried to protect her siblings and all these women were determined to protect their own children from the pattern being repeated down the generations.

Jewels, Emm and Heather had made a virtue out of the fact that they had not told anyone as children. They believed that they had made this choice in order to protect other family members, either a parent or siblings. This choice had enabled them to develop a strong sense of themselves as protectors and helpers of others. They all worked in the helping professions. Jewels believed that she had 'been given a purpose in life that I never had before' to help other victims heal.

The victim narrative can be seen as a personally and socially coherent narrative. This is a narrative form in which things initially go well for the narrator and then suddenly take a dramatic turn for the worse. In the last 20 years victim narratives have, to a large extent, been replaced by survivor narratives.[24] The survivor narrative is now the preferred cultural narrative in the sense that it portrays a young person, usually a woman, who has overcome childhood adversity and has been transformed in the process into a better person. It is a narrative form in which things initially go badly, and then take a dramatic turn for the better. It can also be described as a heroic quest narrative, in the course of which the phoenix rises from the ashes. In this study, it could be seen as the missing narrative of the heroine as opposed to the hero,[25] since all those telling this narrative were women.

NARRATIVE OF JUSTICE AT ANY COST

Three women who had incestuous childhood experiences told *narratives of justice at any cost*. Two of them had tried to tell adults what was happening to them as children and had not been believed. As adults they all made a report about their victimisers to the police, despite the cost to them personally in terms of loss of connection with their families. They were proud of what they had achieved and wanted to protect future generations of children from suffering in the way that they had suffered. They had torn up or burned the worn and stained tapestries of childhood and had woven new ones as adults that contained emblems of justice and advocacy for others.

These women described the grooming process particularly well, although this process was evident in many of the other narratives as well. Perhaps they were able to identify the grooming process, because they had all chosen to report their relatives and had received therapy as a result. This may have helped them to see the actions of the adult for what they were – highly manipulative and exploitative. They also described the way in which the grooming process began with positive reinforcement and moved to threats of various kinds if they withdrew their cooperation in any way.

Seeking justice to protect future generations

Karen, Tina and Jane felt good about themselves for trying to take on their victimisers through the court system, even though it had been at considerable personal expense in terms of their relationships with their families. They had chosen to tell the police as adults and had sought justice for themselves. Not being believed or being punished as children may have strengthened their resolve to do this. They also wanted to break the cycle of abuse within their families and protect their own children from being maltreated. They experienced 'the family's betrayal as actually more painful' than the sexual abuse.

From an attachment theory perspective, we know that if children experience protection from their main caregivers they can internalise the role of protecting others, and will develop the ability to protect themselves. By contrast, children who have been abused often don't know how to protect themselves or others.[26] They don't develop a sense of what it means to protect others and don't have clear boundaries around issues such as touch. However, these women seem to have understood the importance of their roles as protectors of others and were striving for justice and safety for future generations. They used this as the basis for the construction of a positive and resilient narrative about their experiences.

Karen, Tina and Jane chose to break the cycle of abuse within their families, partly in order to protect other children. As Tina put it, 'I didn't want him near my daughter.' This decision cost them all dearly. They all found it necessary to cut off all contact with their families eventually. This was not an easy choice to make and not one that they made lightly, but they knew that it was the right decision for them.

NARRATIVE OF REMAINING DEFIANT

These defiant narratives have appeared less frequently in the literature which is based mainly on research conducted with clinical samples of child sexual abuse survivors who, by definition, accept the role of *survivor*. These men and women were different from those normally studied in that many of them had never attended therapy and they did not identify themselves as victims or survivors of child sexual abuse. They rejected being stereotyped, and longed to be seen as normal. This was not an ethereal *narrative of remaining defiant*, but an earthy narrative told in a down-to-earth manner.

Those telling *narratives of remaining defiant* had thrown away most of the tapestry of childhood and had rewoven a new one. They had incorporated their childhood experiences as a small but inevitable part of life's rich tapestry into the new design, but not as the main focus. They did not want to be reminded of their childhood experiences, refused to dwell on them, and would only refer to them if they felt it would be helpful to other people. This was partly as a result of a strong desire not to be labelled in any way and partly as a result of a 'determinedness to be normal' (Diana). The youngest, Belinda, did not want people 'to think any less of me, or to judge me, or to think that I might become a perpetrator'.

Not a victim or a survivor

These men and women also grew up in abusive environments and had internalised negative messages about themselves, although they seemed more likely to express their anger outwardly through aggressive behaviour towards others. For example, Diana still saw herself as in some ways responsible for being raped and described herself as 'just a silly little girl that got herself into some silly situations [chuckles] that could have cost her life'. However, she also experienced her own sexual power during this incident and declared that 'in that moment I didn't see myself as a victim. I saw myself as being in a position of power.' As an adult she was able to feel empathy and forgiveness towards her rapists.

These men and women wanted to be seen as normal, and battled through many difficulties in their adolescence and early adulthood. For example, Will resisted the idea that 'you've been dirtied by this, you've been broken by this.' They fought against the system in adolescence and young adulthood and adopted a tough exterior. Norm lived with a group of hustlers, Rod joined a skinhead gang and then a bikie gang, Will went to jail, and Diana carried a knife. Some of this behaviour could be described as hypermasculine.[27] Rod believed that he 'dealt with it as a man should', admitted that he 'saw women as sexual objects, to be used and abused' and 'vented all my anger and rage' on homosexuals. However, they had all come through this difficult period to live satisfying lives.

These men and women had moved to a position of not being defined by their childhood maltreatment and some, like Belinda, achieved this in a relatively short time period. They had similar sorts of struggles to others such as feelings of low self-esteem, an inability to trust others, and difficulty in maintaining strong relationships, and yet they transcended these problems, often by taking a spiritual path. They believed that both victim and survivor identities were limiting and potentially stigmatising and rejected both these discourses. They preferred to believe that they were greater than the sum of their childhood experiences.

Spirituality and helping others

A unifying theme in these narratives was that of spirituality, but of a robust nature. These men and women had transcended the difficult experiences in their early lives by choosing to put their faith in a source of power beyond themselves.[28] They believed that their healing had come through a relationship with their Higher Power and through increased empathy for the suffering of others.

Diana, Belinda and Will were all regular churchgoers and actively involved in ministry of various kinds. Diana had a strong faith and demonstrated a practical Christianity by working with drug addicts and alcoholics within her church community. She would invite people into her home to live if they needed somewhere to stay. Belinda described the loss of her relationship with her abusive stepfather as 'a bit of a hole in your soul' which she had managed to fill through being active in her church community. She had gone out on a limb to help other people, including a young woman who had been raped in the small country town where she lived.

Will had no time for people who played what he saw as the 'role of the victim' and hated the focus that the media placed on the 'so-called victim'. He had experienced suffering and, as a result, didn't want to cause suffering in others. After his conversion to Christianity, he had travelled around the country paying back the money that he had stolen from people. He put his beliefs into practice and expected others to do so. As he said: 'If you've been betrayed, you *know* what it is to betray.'

Rod and Norm both attributed the start of their journey through their childhood experiences to contact with Christian organisations. Rod had broken silence first with a member of a Christian motorcycle club and Norm had become a member of Alcoholics Anonymous as an important part of his recovery process. Hence the interwoven themes in *narratives of remaining defiant* were of experiencing great difficulty in childhood through to early adulthood, rebelling and conforming at the same time, refusing to be labelled as a victim or a survivor, and finding a sense of self through service to others.

SUMMARY

Key points
- Both men and women were able to construct resilient self-narratives following childhood sexual experiences.
- The *narrative of normal sexual development* was told by two people who believed that they were unharmed and un-traumatised by their experiences.
- The *narrative of a silence recently broken* was told by men and women who were not traumatised by their experiences, were asymptomatic as children and had been able to use avoidant coping mechanisms successfully. However, they had recently started to wonder if their childhood experiences had affected their ability to create satisfying sexual relationships.
- The *narrative of the need to remember and the need to forget* was told by men and women who were still struggling with the impact of their childhood sexual experiences and remained fragile. They embraced a social identity as victims and demonstrated the least resilience at this stage in their recovery. Hopefully in future they will be able to develop a more resilient narrative.

- The *narrative of protecting and helping others* was told by women who saw themselves as survivors and who valued their role as protectors, even though this didn't involve speaking out about child sexual abuse.
- The *narrative of justice at any cost* was told by women who had been willing to sacrifice their connection with their families in order to bring their victimisers to justice, thereby protecting future generations of children.
- The *narrative of remaining defiant* was a resilient narrative of transcending and overcoming childhood adversity and refusing to accept a stigmatised identity as a survivor of child sexual abuse or to be defined by child maltreatment.
- Despite experiencing childhood adversity, these men and women were able to develop *narratives of resilience* to explain their lives and their choices to themselves and others.

In this chapter I have drawn together the threads of the stories I heard. By examining each of the six main narratives told, I have reconstructed the differing ways in which people have developed resilient narratives. In the following chapter I will discuss gender differences in relation to the development of narratives of resilience and the impact of the wider system on this process. In particular I will examine the impact of the changing social environment and the family environment, and gender differences in disclosure.

Gender differences in the development of narratives of resilience and disclosure

INTRODUCTION

Chapter aims

- Determine the extent to which these resilient narratives are influenced by the social discourse of the times.
- Describe how this process of developing a resilient narrative takes place in the context of the family, whether it is functional or dysfunctional, and how it might be influenced by gender.
- Examine the importance of bearing witness and speaking out against injustice compared with keeping silent and protecting others.
- Discuss the similarities and differences between the genders in relation to disclosure.
- Explore the ways in which the social construction of gender affects narrative construction.
- Consider the difference between heterosexual and homosexual experiences in childhood.
- Examine possible reasons why some men and women move from victim to victimiser.

This chapter examines the impact of changing social constructions around the victim, survivor and child maltreatment discourses on these narratives. The focus is on the family environment and the wider social context and how both these impact on people's ability to generate a resilient narrative. Gender similarities and differences in relation to both disclosure and narrative development are explored.

THE IMPACT OF FAMILY CONTEXT ON NARRATIVE DEVELOPMENT

The family context is widely recognised as important for a child's development. Positive family attributes support the child's development of resilience and adaptive capabilities and can act as protective factors that strengthen the buffering process.[1] The quality and the nature of both peer and family relationships appear to protect children who have had childhood sexual experiences from developing adjustment difficulties or psychiatric disorders in late adolescence. Greater support needs to be given to parents living in disadvantaged families, in order to foster greater resilience in potentially vulnerable children.

Family protective and risk factors

The family environments in which these men and women found themselves affected their ability to tell resilient narratives about themselves. In many ways these families could not provide the protective factors that would help them to thrive and develop despite adversity.[2] As a result, many struggled in childhood, adolescence and early adulthood and had to rely on their individual characteristics and on the wider social environment for sources of support.[3]

In this study, those telling *narratives of normal sexual development* and *narratives of a silence recently broken* were the least likely to have severely damaged relationships within their families, and were the least likely to have sought out the support of others through therapy. Most of the other men and women experienced varying degrees of child maltreatment and socioeconomic deprivation, had alcoholic parents, developed poor attachment relationships within the family and were often forced to live with their victimiser. They also tended to have poor attachment relationships with the non-abusing parent and came from chaotic families in which all forms of child maltreatment were common.

Socioeconomic deprivation is known to be a risk factor in families where the adults are investigated for maltreatment of their children.[4] The impact of the family context was significant for many of the men and women interviewed in this study. About half of them experienced impoverished childhoods and most experienced more than one form of child maltreatment.[5] Poverty was mentioned explicitly by three people but was hinted at by six more who had all experienced various forms of deprivation in childhood. Four women described feeling isolated from other people and trapped within the family as they grew up in rural areas. Half the men grew up in boarding schools, institutions or with other family members.

Some studies suggest that children whose parents have low levels of education, or a history of psychiatric illness, drug or alcohol use or childhood abuse, are more likely to live in families that are investigated for child maltreatment.[6] In this study poverty was often exacerbated by parental alcohol abuse leading to chaotic family life. One-third of these men and women grew up in families where one caregiver was an alcoholic and over half of them grew up in families where domestic violence and physical abuse was common. Heather described her role as the person that tried to calm her drunken father when he became angry: 'If I could smooth him over, or divert him or something like that, then the violence would dissipate.' Half of the women experienced acts of cruelty at the hands of their fathers or at the hands of their mothers. Only Bert and Angelo reported no form of child maltreatment at home and Jim experienced physical abuse only. Otherwise frequent child maltreatment was the norm at home and impacted on their ability to develop positive self-narratives as children.

Sexual abuse was an intergenerational issue in many of these families and particularly among those telling *narratives of forgetting and remembering, protecting and helping others or justice at any cost.* Over half the women believed that their mothers had been sexually abused as children, and two-thirds believed that their siblings had also been sexually abused, although not necessarily by the same adult. Rod and Colin believed that their victimisers had also been sexually abused as children, although this was not offered as an excuse for their behaviour in any way.

For many, the family context in which they grew up was both chaotic and unsupportive. As Norm said, 'it seemed like there was chaos wherever I was'. This was probably less true for those telling *narratives of normal sexual development* or *narratives of a silence recently broken.* However, most others did not receive the care and attention that they needed as children. They had little support from family members and were unable to discuss events or receive reassurance that they were not in the wrong themselves. In a sense, the chaotic family environment limited the narratives that were available to them, and may even had added to the trauma of their childhood sexual experiences and to the potential for the transmission of risk to the next generation.

Many of those interviewed believed that their own children had a higher risk of being sexually abused and described feeling very protective towards them. Diana was convinced that her sons were just as at risk as a daughter would be because 'I've no trust in men'. Tina described her concern about the way in which her daughter was being drawn into the family against her will. 'It's almost like you are being groomed by the family.' This was one of the reasons that Tina and others felt the need to cut off contact with their families, in order to break this intergenerational pattern of behaviour even though her relatives 'wanted to keep the family intact . . . this fabulous family'.

Poor attachment within the family

Given these family contexts, it was difficult for these men and women to develop the necessary attachment bonds with their parents.[7] Only Diana claimed to be close to her mother at the time of the interview, saying, 'I ring her almost every day but I would never, ever tell her this story because she wouldn't cope with it.' Those telling *narratives of normal sexual development* or *narratives of a silence recently broken* were more likely than others to have better relationships with family members. They felt protective towards one or both parents, not wishing them to know about their childhood experiences. Apart from Peter, they had childhood sexual experiences with non-family members and, perhaps as a result, found it easier to maintain contact and feel protective towards their parents than those who had childhood sexual experiences within the family.

However, in this study 12 out of 22 men and women lived in the same home as the adults with whom they had sexual contact, which may be over-representative of those who have been sexually abused by family members.[8] Family relationships are known to be highly complex for those people who have experienced incest in childhood. Several of these men and women described having enmeshed relationships with the parent with whom they had early sexual contact. Some came from sexually permissive family backgrounds which left them feeling very confused and with no real sense of right or wrong around this sexual contact. Others came from sexually repressive, religious family backgrounds. When Leo tried to tell his Catholic mother what had happened to him, 'all she saw was the badness in it' and, by implication, in Leo himself.

Although it is theoretically possible for children to create a secure attachment with a non-abusive parent while forming an insecure attachment with an abusive parent,[9] there was little evidence of strong attachments with non-abusive parents surviving into adulthood. Two-thirds of the women had felt the need to cut off all contact with their mothers as adults because of their lack of protective behaviour towards their daughters. Karen made this decision when she left home. 'From when I was 18, I didn't have a father or a mother any more.' Jewels felt unable to trust men or women because 'my mother abandoned me, she allowed it to happen. So I felt as though she betrayed me and I felt as though I was betrayed by men, too.'

Four women were still struggling with ongoing conflict in their relationships with their mothers. The relationship with one parent had a bearing on the relationship with the other. For example, Emm had a distant relationship with her mother who was physically cruel and emotionally distant. She described physical contact with her mother as 'like hugging a block of ice'. Partly as a result of this she needed to be close to her father and she 'liked being close to Dad, that's the most painful thing'. If one parent was abusive, the need for a close bond with the other parent perhaps heightened the feelings of loss or betrayal when this parent failed to live up to expectations.

THE IMPACT OF THE WIDER SOCIAL SYSTEM

The discourse around child sexual abuse has changed and developed over time and has influenced the social acceptability or otherwise of certain narratives. Driven by the feminist agenda in the 1970s and 1980s, child sexual abuse was named publicly as a crime against women and children.[10] Paedophiles were exposed by their victims and sent to jail. Incest was discussed more openly, although fear of paedophilia and sensationalised stories were the main focus for the Australian media.[11] Having been a hidden discourse for many years, it became socially acceptable to discuss being a victim or, preferably, a survivor of child sexual abuse. The survivor discourse became popular, particularly among women, although less so among men.

After the millennium when this study was conducted, some of the men and women interviewed were comfortable adopting the mantle of the victim or the survivor, whereas others vehemently rejected what they saw as a stigmatising discourse. Many struggled with the issue of whether or not to speak out about their experiences. If they chose to speak out, they needed to be prepared to accept the label of victim or survivor of child sexual abuse – whether or not this label fitted the way that they themselves viewed their childhood experiences. But if they chose to keep silent in order to protect their reputation and that of their family, they could be accused of protecting the victimiser and failing to protect other children.

The need to bear witness and speak out against injustice

In Australia, the national saying for honouring soldiers who are killed in action is 'lest we forget'. There is a powerful social discourse around the need to remember, which is often finely balanced against the individual's need to forget. Following trauma, this tension is particularly potent and can be seen particularly in the literature relating to human atrocities. The need to remember and to find a collective voice is often linked to the need to bear witness and to prevent similar occurrences from happening in the future.[12] Speaking out about horrific events, such as the Holocaust, helps survivors to develop a shared cultural history and to achieve a collective acceptance of the reality of events. However, the need to forget and to move forward in life or the desire to protect the next generation from the pain and anguish that has been endured is equally strong. This tension is also found in the grief literature between theorists that advocate the importance of maintaining a *continuing bond* with the deceased, and those that advocate *letting go* or saying goodbye in order to move on with life.[13]

Childhood sexual experiences with adults may differ from atrocities that affect a particular cultural group, in that talking about such events is often met with denial rather than validation within the family. In cases of severe trauma, individuals can also be silenced through amnesia. This may go some way towards explaining the popularity of group therapy among some survivors who may yearn for the validation of their experiences and the recognition afforded by membership of a group.

Different people dealt with the tension between the need to bear witness and the need to move forward with life in different ways and there may be an underlying development process in operation. Those telling *narratives of a silence recently broken* for many years privileged the need to forget and move forward over the need to bear witness. As time went by, and the media discussion of the impact of child sexual abuse on its victims increased, they slowly began to question their own narratives. Peter started to question 'why are all these people getting so upset about this?' when he was not upset himself. Jim came to the realisation that 'I've never really put it down.' They began to see possible connections between their childhood sexual experiences and ongoing difficulties in their intimate lives.

Although the increased media attention enabled people to speak out about abuse, it also had some negative aspects with victim and survivor stories becoming appropriated and exploited by the media. As more and more celebrities and public figures acknowledged that they had experienced child sexual abuse, and discussed the terrible impact that it had on their lives, it became harder for those telling *narratives of normal sexual development* or *narratives of a silence recently broken* or to maintain that they had not been affected in any way by their experiences. Bert described being reluctant to talk to close friends about his experiences because 'I'm afraid of their reaction because I don't think that I've been traumatised by this event'. He knew that this was a socially unacceptable thing to say in public, for fear of being labelled a child abuser, a homosexual or even a paedophile. While maintaining these narratives in private, he and others felt silenced publicly by their socially dysfunctional narratives.

While they believed that they made the right choice in remaining silent, they came to realise that there was a cost associated with this choice. They had to withstand the increasing pressure placed on them in the current social climate to tell their stories in the form of a moral tale.[14] They knew that 'people say it's always good to talk about things that troubled you.' They also questioned whether or not they should have told someone about their experiences in order to protect other children. For example, Peter asked himself 'Has he abused somebody else because I didn't spill the beans?' He experienced strong feelings of guilt as a result.

Being silenced or choosing silence

Those telling *narratives of the need to remember and the need to forget, protecting and helping others,* or *justice at any cost* had been silenced as children and adolescents, sometimes through a process of amnesia. They had all found a voice in adulthood, sometimes through the painful process of recovering memories of childhood maltreatment. There was a sense in which some of them felt silenced whereas others believed that they had chosen silence in order to protect others. Karen described the relief of telling the police 'this secret that's been held in for so long. I've told somebody that's going to do something about it', whereas Emm knew that 'it would have been devastating as a child to put this together' and that maintaining silence had been a mechanism of self-protection. Some accepted a sense of themselves as victims, whereas others were moving towards seeing themselves as survivors. Either way, the process involved speaking, in therapy and elsewhere, about what had happened to them as children.

For those telling *narratives of remaining defiant,* their reluctance to adopt the identity as a victim or a survivor meant that they were less keen to talk about their experiences publicly or to risk being categorised by others in any way. However, they were perfectly willing to do so if they believed that it would be helpful to others. The context appeared to dictate their behaviour.

GENDER SIMILARITIES AND DIFFERENCES IN DISCLOSURE

It is far more common for children not to make a disclosure than it is for them to make a disclosure[15] and this may be intentional for some children.[16] As can be seen from these narratives, children often have good reason to be fearful about the possible consequences of disclosure which can be negative for them and for their families. Without a supportive family environment, they are unlikely to feel safe enough to discuss their childhood sexual experiences.[17] Of course, it is difficult for a child to have control over what happens or to have a complete understanding of the possible consequences of a disclosure being made, and sometimes someone else will make a report against their wishes. In this study, only four people made a disclosure to a relative in childhood, usually their mothers, and one had a disclosure made on her behalf by her stepmother.

Despite difficulties, these men and women did gradually decide to talk to other people about their childhood sexual experiences as they became adults. This supports the concept of disclosure as a developmental process.[18] As adults, they had more control over the process and more understanding of the likely consequences for members of the family. Five made *purposeful disclosures* to the police, in the hope of breaking the cycle of abuse and seeking justice. A further five told their families what had happened to them, despite the inevitable negative consequences of doing so. But 12 people made *selective disclosures* only, preferring to continue to protect either themselves or their families from full knowledge of what had happened to them as children. These attempts to protect their families may have been misguided.[19] Nine told their intimate partners or their friends, two told their therapists during a process of recovering memories and one told the researcher. Some had come to regret not making a report to the police earlier and felt guilty about failing to protect other children from abuse.

Fear, shame and self-blame as inhibitors to disclosure

The main inhibitors to disclosure were fear, shame and self-blame. Many of these adults felt fearful as children, with some justification. Many of them grew up in situations of relative poverty, in fear-ridden families that were ruled by violent men. The abuse of alcohol added to this volatile mix to ensure that their fears were well founded. Some were deliberately frightened by their victimisers and were threatened with being punished if they told anyone what was happening within the family. Fear was an entirely appropriate response and explains why many children did not tell anyone. They were afraid that they wouldn't be believed, afraid that they would be punished and, perhaps more importantly, afraid of the negative consequences for other members of the family that they long to protect. Fortunately for most, the level of fear diminished once they were more in control of their own destiny as adults.

Shame acted as a powerful inhibitor, especially for the men interviewed. Once they grew into adolescence and began to understand the homosexual nature of their childhood experiences, they felt a great deal of shame and feared exposure for that reason. Many also took on a sense of self-blame and responsibility for what was happening to them. They believed that they should have been able to prevent it or to stop it from happening, particularly as they grew older. This sense of shame did not diminish, perhaps because it was sanctioned by societal views that men should not be victims of child sexual abuse and that homosexuality is problematic.

Fear a stronger inhibitor for girls, shame for boys

Those adults that reported feeling scared or ashamed as children or who tended to blame themselves for what happened were less likely to tell anyone as children or as adults. People of both sexes tended to attribute blame to themselves rather than to their victimiser, but women were more likely to admit to being scared in childhood, and men were more likely to admit to feeling ashamed of what had happened to them as children. This may have helped women to make *purposeful disclosures* in adulthood and may have led to men continuing to making *selective disclosures* only. The current literature suggests that men often have homophobic responses to child sexual abuse and fear that 'homosexuality was either the cause or effect of the abuse'.[20] A third concern emerged – men did not want to be labelled as homosexual by others.

Purposeful disclosures by women, selective disclosures by men

Four out of five of those who tried to tell someone as children were women and nine out of 10 who chose to tell either the police or their families as adults were women. *Purposeful disclosure* was much more common among women than men as adults, with nine out of 13 women making purposeful disclosures compared to one out of nine men. *Selective disclosure* was much more common in adulthood among men, with eight out of nine men making *selective disclosures* and only four out of 13 women doing so.

This may partly relate to the level of shame experienced by these men. It may also relate to the way in which women are socialised to seek help whereas men find it more difficult to acknowledge their vulnerability and need for help. I believe that women are more supported by society in the role of victim and are therefore more able to acknowledge this and to seek social support.

GENDER SIMILARITIES AND DIFFERENCES IN NARRATIVE CONSTRUCTION

There is a need to understand gender similarities and differences in relation to childhood sexual experiences. One of the similarities is that both genders developed resilient narratives.

Developing a resilient narrative despite difficulties with intimacy

There are many different resilient narratives that people tell themselves and others about their childhood sexual experiences. Some are private narratives of not being badly affected, of maintaining a dignified silence in order to protect other family members from a painful reality, of struggling with forgetting and remembering, or of protecting siblings. Other resilient narratives are more public in nature and describe the ways in which people, many of them women, have overcome or transcended their childhood maltreatment, have told their families despite severe consequences, have campaigned against child sexual abuse, or have reported their victimisers to the police.

These narratives are more complex in nature than the popular survivor discourse. As adults, these men and women weighed up the advantages of telling versus the ongoing benefits of not telling. They weighed up the consequences, not only for themselves but for other family members, other potential victims and society in general. Some opted for *purposeful disclosure*, but this was still easier for women than for men. Others opted for *selective disclosure*, in order to continue to protect others. And there will be many other people that were, by definition, excluded from this study who choose non-disclosure even as adults.

Qualitative studies have suggested that men and women who are survivors of child sexual abuse have difficulty forming and maintaining intimate and satisfying sexual relationships. Trust was a big issue for many of these men and women.[21] One of the most commonly reported ways in which they believed that they had been impacted by their childhood sexual experiences was in their intimate relationships. For example, as adolescents and young adults half of these men and women found themselves having non-committed sex with multiple partners. However, this didn't stop the development of narratives of resilience.

Culturally sanctioned and supported role for women as victims

The social construction of victimhood as a feminine concept appeared to have some positive aspects for women. Women seemed to be more able than men to be transformed by their childhood sexual experiences in a positive manner. Perhaps because it was more socially acceptable for women to be victims, it was also easier for them to talk about their experiences publicly and to seek out the support that they needed.

Many of these women were socially conditioned to believe that they should subjugate their own needs and desires in order to maintain relationships with others.[22] This led them to take responsibility for what happened to them in their childhood and to turn their anger inwards. There were many examples of women, like Jewels, who would 'take on the blame for everything' including what had happened to them as children. Many of these women took on the role of protector of others, like Belinda, by 'looking after everybody else but yourself,' at the expense of their own relationship needs. However, for some women this role was a positive one. Overall these women were probably more successful than the men interviewed at moving on from their childhood experiences and mobilising support.

Although the women described feeling inferior to men and to blaming themselves when they were younger, many had overcome this as adults. They had become powerful women in their own right. They believed that this had occurred partly as a result of working through their childhood sexual experiences, particularly the eight women telling *narratives of protecting and helping others, justice at any cost or remaining defiant.* They had either become protective of others through their work or had mobilised their anger into taking action.

Beyond the gender stereotypes

Feminists have argued that women have been stereotypically divided into either Madonnas or whores,[23] good girls who are virgins or bad girls who are sexually active.[24] Within this book both these extremes of behaviour were evident, with many women describing themselves in a derogatory manner because they had non-committed sex with men at certain stages of their lives. Others, like Tina, described themselves as 'avoiding boys when I was growing up' or as being sexually timid or withdrawn. However, this dichotomous view of women as 'sluts' or 'prudes' was an oversimplification, given the complexity of the situations that they had faced as young girls. For some women who had frequent non-committed sex with men there were serious consequences to their behaviour. For example, Diana became pregnant at 15 and had to leave school and have her child adopted, Karen had a termination at 16 and Sylvia had several terminations.

Although the dominant cultural image of femininity is that of a selfless woman who is subservient to men,[25] half the women interviewed did not behave in stereotypically feminine ways or willingly accept male domination.

For example, Greta saw herself as in control of her childhood sexual experiences and was 'a bit proud' of how she handled herself. Hope, the anti-serial child rapist campaigner, and Diana and Belinda expressed a lot of anger during the interview. Diana defiantly declared that 'I'd rather that people think I'm a tart than a victim.'

Some women were better at mobilising their anger and placing the blame on their victimisers than others.[26] Three women used their own strengths and resources to seek justice without any support from their families. Karen was proud of the fact that 'I done the right thing, by myself.' They demonstrated that women are often better than men at finding strengths from within in order to overcome childhood adversity.[27] None of the men in the study had done this. They seemed trapped by stereotypical societal expectations of the adult male.

Victimisers are constructed as male

The men interviewed seemed to be strongly influenced by societal beliefs about masculinity, often becoming aggressive or stoical about their childhood experiences. They described experiencing non-relational sex and rarely recognised this as a possible form of re-victimisation or re-enactment of their childhood experiences. They were concerned that homosexuality could be the cause or effect of their homosexual encounters in childhood and were also fearful of being labelled as homosexual. It was difficult to talk about their childhood sexual experiences, whether they were heterosexual or homosexual experiences.

The social construction of victimisers as male and the concept of intergenerational patterns of abuse created difficulties for these men. If they spoke out about their experiences, they were fearful about being labelled as either homosexual or potential victimisers themselves. This made it harder for them to reach out for help, thereby potentially increasing the danger that they might move from victim to victimiser.

Masculinity can be viewed as a rejection of femininity and of dependence.[28] 'For men, the central mechanisms are, arguably, projection and denial. Dependency needs and the associated feelings of rage and destructiveness are experienced as existing in, and are perhaps even elicited from, others.'[29] As a result, society condones 'tough, forceful, and aggressively defensive' behaviour in the Australian male as typical and acceptable.[30] This stereotypical 'Aussie male' behaviour was demonstrated by Rod, who decided that he didn't want anyone to get close to him. Other men also acted aggressively during their adolescence.

On the other hand, there were men like Bert, Angelo and Peter who did not behave in a stereotypically aggressive masculine manner. Rather they tended to demonstrate a masculine stoicism[31] often shown by survivors of childhood sexual abuse. The construction of 'real men' as independent, strong, active and knowing how to avoid problems[32] may have fed into the need for these men to appear to be unaffected by their childhood sexual experiences.

The gender socialisation process can lead men to a focus on sexual conquests and to experience problems with intimacy and non-relational sex.[33] Six out of nine men in this study felt ashamed of what had happened to them. Many of them had experienced difficulties of one kind or another in their intimate lives. Many of these men had times when they had non-committed sex with either men or women or both. They believed that they had been active partners in these encounters and did not see them as a form of re-victimisation. Four out of nine men described having had extramarital affairs.

Lusterman described the repetitive seduction of women as a form of 'retaliation toward the woman who is its object. Don Juanism, then, is an example of gender role dysfunction, abetted by a male ideology that objectifies women, and probably compounded by early familial history'.[34] This description fitted Angelo whose sexual behaviour with women troubled him a great deal. Whether or not the behaviour of these men was normal masculine behaviour, non-relational sex, re-victimisation, or a re-enactment of abuse was difficult to determine. However, it is possible that they experienced constraints on their ability to experience mutually satisfying and intimate experiences with women as a result of adopting a traditionally masculine approach to relationships.[35]

Perhaps these men were pushed to the extreme of their gender repertoire. Some became ultra-masculine and aggressive, whereas others were determined to be 'normal' according to the cultural script in Australia.[36] That meant that they became strong, silent and inviolable. They withdrew from intimacy in relationships and suppressed all memories of abuse, choosing to get on with life rather than to dwell on the past. If their experiences were homosexual in nature, the homophobia that they internalised from the culture may have become exaggerated and impacted on their relationships with other men. They may have found it difficult to move away from this stance, becoming frozen in a cultural stereotype, and may have needed to wait until middle age before moving towards other people in a more meaningful way.

The problem of internalised homophobia for men

Men who have been sexually abused by men often have strong homophobic reactions and can be concerned that these might have been caused by their own hidden homosexuality or that they might become homosexual as a result.[37] In this book several men were fearful that they would be seen or labelled as homosexual if others knew about the event. The stigma of the label of homosexuality was of concern to them. For example, four men admitted to being homophobic and to being fearful that people would find out about their childhood sexual experiences with men. Colin lived in a poor neighbourhood as a child and believed that 'you'd be eaten alive if that sort of thing got out'. They seemed to embrace traditionally masculine behaviours such as being tough and aggressive. There was a great reluctance within these men when young to disclose any information about their childhood sexual experiences, partly for fear of this stigma.[38] Of the men interviewed, only one had tried to tell anyone as a child and only four had told people, other than their partners, as adults. Four had not disclosed their experiences to anyone other than their partners before the interview.

Norm, Leo and Bert were open about their adolescent homosexual experiences but did not believe that their sexuality had been affected by their childhood experiences. Bert said, 'I've sort of got straighter as I've got older,' whereas Norm was comfortable to admit that 'I consider myself sexually ambivalent right now.' As adults, they all rejected the notion that a childhood sexual experience could change their sexuality or cause homosexuality.

The problematic 'Mrs Robinson' narrative

The popular 'Mrs Robinson' story of the seduction of a young boy by an older woman in the movie *The Graduate* can be seen as supporting stereotypical masculine constructs. 'The male victim, having been programmed by movies and other media, may regard a sexual relationship with an older woman as a male fantasy come true.'[39] In this study three men were sexually assaulted by women. None described these relationships as anything like a fantasy, but Angelo certainly feared that other men might say 'you're lucky, you hit the lottery', thereby minimising his experiences. These three men certainly had difficulties in their sexual interactions with women. Angelo could only have sex with women he despised, whereas Norm and Leo described enmeshed relationships with their abusive mothers and complicated sexual relationships with both men and women.

From victim to victimiser

This book does not examine victimisers. However, it was clear that some of these men recognised that they could potentially have become victimisers had things been slightly different. For example, one found himself becoming attracted to teenage girls as a middle-aged man, another described his attraction to young children as an adult as 'such an incredible sense of longing', and a third described trying to have 'penetrating sex' with boys his age when he was an adolescent. The potentially sexually abusive behaviour described by these men resonated with the description of child sexual abuse survivors being unable to feel empathy for the distress of the victim.[40] By contrast Rod's concerns about his own level of violence towards women and Jim's experiences of bondage and discipline with consenting adult women resonated more with the concept of the male survivor turning his own distress into anger and sexual violence.[41]

There is an important gender difference in that men are more likely than women to move from victim to victimiser. This has been linked to patriarchy and issues of male power over women and children,[42] given that child maltreatment has historically been associated with the exercise of positions of power. However, the relational difficulties experienced by survivors of child sexual abuse are similar to those experienced by all men.[43] Given that relational skills are not viewed as traditionally masculine,[44] it is possible to argue that men are more vulnerable to moving from victim to victimiser in part because of the restraints placed on them by traditional masculinity.[45] Perhaps they do not make healing empathic connections with others as easily as women.

One important question that remains to be answered is why the men in this study didn't move from victim to victimiser. According to one man, it was his concern not to damage others in the way that he had been damaged that prevented him from becoming a victimiser. As he said, 'I know what it's like to be hurt as a child and I don't want that to happen to any other kid on my behalf.' This view was echoed by most men and women in this study who wanted to protect children from suffering in the way that they had themselves.

SUMMARY

Key points

- It is remarkable that people who came from dysfunctional family backgrounds were still able to tell *resilient narratives* in adulthood.
- Many of these men and women grew up in relative poverty, living with alcoholic parents in chaotic households, experiencing many forms of child maltreatment, and in situations of intergenerational child sexual abuse. They had poor attachment relationships with their parents and many lived with their victimisers.
- There was resilience to be found in both bearing witness and speaking out against injustice and in remaining silent and protecting others. There was also a cost associated with both courses of action.
- Non-disclosure was far more common than disclosure, which was often associated with its own trauma.
- A supportive family environment was necessary for disclosure to take place in childhood. Unfortunately, this was often missing.
- Fear was a strong inhibitor to disclosure among girls, and shame among boys, whereas both genders experienced self-blame as a barrier to disclosure.
- As adults, women were more likely to make *purposeful disclosures* and men were more likely to make *selective disclosures.*
- Both men and women were able to develop resilient narratives, despite experiencing difficulties with intimacy.
- In some ways, societal beliefs supported women as victims more than

men, since being a victim was a culturally sanctioned role for a woman. Paradoxically, this may have empowered some women to make disclosures and to seek help.

- Men were not expected to be victims of child sexual abuse. Their responses were complicated by issues relating to homophobia and to traditional masculinity, which required them to be either aggressive or stoical about their childhood maltreatment.
- Being sexually abused by a woman had different connotations for a young boy than being sexually abused by a man.
- As a result of these complications, men had more difficulty telling people about their experiences and seeking help. This may also partly explain why more men move from victim to victimiser.

In this chapter I have discussed how people develop resilient narratives over time within difficult family environments, how these narratives change with the changing social context and how they are influenced by gender issues. The final chapter will explore the implications for how we work in therapy with adults who have had childhood sexual experiences, including a 10-step plan for recovery from relational injury. It will also discuss how you can help a loved one, perhaps a family member or a friend, who has had this misfortune themselves. And, finally, it will challenge you to consider how, if at all, your attitudes to this complex topic have been changed by reading this book.

CHAPTER 12

How to heal relational injuries caused by childhood sexual experiences

INTRODUCTION

Chapter aims

- Explain the implications of this research for health professionals working with adults who have had childhood sexual experiences.
- Describe a 10-step recovery plan for adults who have had childhood sexual experiences, whether or not they view these experiences as abusive.
- Explain how to support loved ones who have had, or are currently going through, similar experiences.
- Encourage the reader to review their attitudes towards this complex topic, having read this book.

This book challenges some of the conventional views held about child sexual abuse. By interviewing a broader range of men and women and by inviting them to tell their stories about their childhood sexual experiences with adults, a wider range of narratives emerged. These narratives go beyond the victim and survivor discourses and have implications for theory and practice. I believe that they should be used to inform how clinicians work with the relational injuries that adults often experience following child maltreatment.

In focusing on relational injuries and on resilient narratives, I risk being accused of minimising the impact of child sexual abuse or of supporting paedophilia in some way. This is not my intention. I abhor acts of violence against children or anyone else for that matter. But I believe that there is reason to be hopeful that many children can overcome such potentially damaging experiences in adulthood, by developing resilient narratives about their experiences and by being supported to overcome the relational injuries that they are likely to have sustained in childhood.

RELATIONAL INJURIES

In this section I describe the new knowledge that has emerged about how people cope with their childhood sexual experiences. These contributions to knowledge are wide-ranging and cover the issues of: the relational injuries caused; the importance of gender differences; the developmental difficulties associated with disclosure in childhood; the wide range of functional narratives used; and the limitations of current socially acceptable narratives.

Childhood sexual experiences leading to relational injury

The research underpinning this book challenges the focus on *trauma* in this field and places it, instead, on *relational injury*. The word trauma derives from the Greek word meaning 'wound' but has evolved to mean the physical and psychological response to such a wound or distressing event or series of events. The most crucial influence on the development of a resilient narrative is the extent to which people experience wounds in their relationships, rather than traumatic experiences. Not all have experienced a traumatic event or a traumatic response to a series of events, whereas all are likely to have suffered from relational injuries or the wounds from the damage inflicted on their childhood relationships with adults, often those closest to them.

A common thread that wove between narratives told was that people had difficulty in making and maintaining intimate connections with other people in adulthood. They believed that this difficulty stemmed from their interactions with adults in childhood, where trust was broken and they were left feeling responsible and to blame for what happened.[1] This affected their ability to trust other people, to confide in them, to see themselves through the eyes of others, and to form caring relationships.

Many people experienced the fracturing of relationships within their families, and a sense of betrayal by members of the family. This left them vulnerable to re-victimisation and they frequently experienced further relationship problems in adolescence and early adulthood, often exacerbated by their own behaviour. Even those telling a *narrative of a silence recently broken* who believed that their childhood sexual experiences had not affected them were beginning to question whether or not they had, after all, been affected in terms of their ability to experience intimate connections with others.

It is possible to conceptualise the issue of child sexual abuse in terms of relational injury. From this perspective, the central difficulty for children is that they experience a *deep wound within a close relationship*. This wound is often sexual, physical and psychological. This wound destroys the child's trust in others and creates difficulties in other close bonds. Of course, this relational injury may inform the level of trauma experienced by the child or adolescent, who may or may not go on to develop symptoms of post-traumatic stress disorder. However, the core issue here is not the traumatic experience but the damage done to the child's ability to connect closely with others.[2] For example, those telling a *narrative of normal sexual development* or *a silence recently broken* did not describe their experiences as traumatic but now believe that they did sustain relational injuries of some kind.

The severity of the relational injury caused by childhood sexual experience with an adult may be the crucial factor, rather than the level of trauma experienced by the child or adolescent. The experience of trauma may be influenced by the level of relational injury experienced, rather than the other way round. This helps to explain why those men and women telling a *narrative of normal sexual development* or *a narrative of a silence recently broken* were able to demonstrate resilience, which has a relational aspect, in the face of adversity. Their childhood sexual experiences were slightly less severe and more likely to be with non-family members, started slightly later into adolescence, and their family relationships were slightly less dysfunctional than for others. As a result, they were able to avoid severe relational injuries and were therefore able to maintain a stronger sense of themselves as successful people, despite their childhood sexual experiences. They still view their experiences as non-traumatic today.

This is not an entirely new idea and was embedded in Erickson's (1963) work of psychosocial stages of development and Bowlby's work on affectional bonds.[3] Finkelhor's[4] four traumagenic dynamics of sexual abuse (traumatic sexualisation, betrayal, stigmatisation and powerlessness) can all be seen as causing difficulties in the formation of new relationships. The early sexualisation of the child leads to further non-relational sexual acts that can lead to re-victimisation, thereby perpetuating relational injuries. Betrayal, stigmatisation and powerlessness all cause relational problems. Herman[5] saw disempowerment and disconnection as central issues in trauma work, recognised the primary importance of the damage done to relationships in terms of attachment theory and argued that the recovery process takes place in the context of a healing relationship. Robb also argued that trauma is a relational injury.[6]

The concept of trauma has become such a dominant theoretical concept in this field that it has overshadowed the concept of relational injury. Fleming and Mullen focused more on relationship issues when they developed a social and developmental model for child sexual abuse.[7] They saw mental health problems associated with child sexual abuse as second-order effects and proposed that the primary damage, especially in less severe cases, was to the child's development of trust, a sense of agency, a relational ability to be intimate with others, and to their sexuality. This research supports a model of relational injury, particularly in less severe cases, which has implications for clinicians working in this field. There are also some important gender differences with regard to relational injury caused by childhood sexual experiences.

Gender differences in relational injury

The research findings discussed in this book suggest important gender differences in child sexual abuse. Seeing the issue as one of relational injury goes some way to explaining the important gender differences in this field. Boys are far less likely than girls to disclose their childhood sexual experiences with adults and are far more likely to go on to become victimisers of others, even though most do not. If the injury is a relational one, the damage may be more severe for boys than for girls. Given that in general boys do not value relationships in the same way that girls do, have fewer relational skills and are restricted emotionally, they may find it even harder than girls to recover from child sexual abuse and experience more psychiatric symptoms in adulthood.[8] Given their reluctance to disclose their experiences, they have fewer options available to them than girls and are generally less likely to seek help.

Gender differences in response to childhood sexual experiences need to be better understood by health professionals, as well as the impact of the social construction of gender. Men who have had childhood sexual experiences can be torn between their desire to accept traditional masculine roles, and the risk they take of being labelled as effeminate if they reveal their victim status. Men may go on to experience even greater difficulties than women with intimate relationships, non-relational sex, aggressive behaviour and fear of being labelled as homosexual. However, it should be noted that this research does not speak to the issue of girls having homosexual experiences because the sample did not include any women who had childhood sexual experiences with women.

In general, men are stereotypically viewed as victimisers and women as victims. In some ways this positioning has helped women to be more open about their experiences and to move out of the victim role and into the survivor role. It may have exacerbated the difficulties for men who want to avoid being labelled as weak and emasculated, homosexual or as potential paedophiles. Whether or not their childhood sexual experiences were with men or women, men have greater difficulty in disclosing that they have been sexually abused as children. In fact, disclosure is developmentally difficult for children of both genders.

The developmental difficulty of disclosure in childhood

Disclosure is seen as vital by health professionals and by those involved in criminal justice, for obvious reasons. If the child or adult does not tell anyone then the abuse will continue, victimisers cannot be identified and be held responsible for their actions and the recovery process cannot begin. However, disclosure is a difficult process[9] and is developmentally demanding for children. There are so many hurdles for the child to overcome in order to make a disclosure. The barriers to disclosure that emerged included the unsupportive family context and the level of fear, shame or self-blame experienced by the child. There were additional barriers of stigma and prejudice to be overcome when the experience was homosexual in nature and disclosure proved to be even more difficult for men than for women.

This study adds to the evidence that disclosure is a difficult process for children and adults to go through[10] and that it has the potential to create problems within families.[11] Most people didn't tell as children and often delayed telling until adulthood. They believed that they had made the right decision not to tell and would do the same again. Many made a positive out of this decision and developed a sense of themselves as protecting other family members by their actions. It was only recently that those telling a *narrative of a silence recently broken* had started to question whether their decision not to tell might have resulted in other children being harmed, even though it protected their own families from distress. Some men and women were still choosing to protect family members by not telling them what happened, even well into adulthood.

Even though they believed that they had made the right decision within their particular family context not to tell, they also believed that it was better for other children if they could tell someone. In other words, they believed that children should live in a loving environment where disclosure was possible. However, this was not the environment that most of them had experienced as children and, for the five men and women that had tried to tell, the situation did not significantly improve afterwards. The preconditions for disclosure simply did not exist for most of them. These preconditions include a high level of trust within the family, the expectation that the adult would believe the child's version of events, and the belief that no one in the family would be harmed as a result of the disclosure.

Resilient narratives of overcoming relational injuries

Most people found resilient narratives to help them to view and live with their childhood experiences. Those telling a *narrative of normal sexual development* or *a narrative of a silence recently broken* believed for many years that they had not been negatively affected by their experiences. This could be seen as an avoidant coping mechanism of some kind. Avoidant coping works well in situations where the relational injury is less severe and where the child has reasonably good relationships within the family. This is supported by the way in which avoidant coping mechanisms used by these men and women did not indicate serious psychopathology.

Narrative therapy[12] offers a way to view such coping mechanisms as an act of resistance by the child when facing challenging circumstances. The therapist and the client deconstruct the oppressive narrative and examine the social, cultural and historical context that influenced the original creation of the narrative, and co-construct an alternative narrative that is emancipatory.[13] For example, one man kept silent about his childhood sexual experiences with an older cousin because he accepted the oppressive narrative that it was his fault and that *they* would get into trouble if anyone knew. As an adult, a therapist could help him to understand that his cousin manipulated him into believing this. He might also come to see that his fear of his father's violent reaction, his concern that his mother would not believe him and his own internalised homophobia also influenced his decision not to tell anyone as a child. Together they would work out the influence of the social restraints of that time and reinterpret his decision not to tell.

The challenge with taking a narrative approach is that both the therapist and the client may come to see narratives in a dichotomous way, as either 'bad' or 'good'.[14] Some therapists and clients might view a *narrative of normal sexual development* or *a narrative of a silence recently broken* as 'bad' narratives because they enabled the person telling them to deny the reality of their childhood experiences and the victimiser to escape the consequences. Others might view a *narrative of the need to remember and the need to forget* as a 'bad' narrative similar to that of the damaged victim, and *narratives of protecting and helping others* or *justice at any cost* as 'good' because of their similarities to the socially acceptable, heroic survivor narrative. The central thrust of this book is that all these narratives appeared to be helpful to those telling them at the time of the interview. However, only some of these narratives are currently socially acceptable.

Resilient narratives beyond the victim and survivor discourses

This book adds evidence to the growing body of knowledge about the potentially limiting impact of the victim and survivor discourses. Half of the men and women in this study didn't relate to either of these discourses. Those telling a *narrative of remaining defiant* didn't want their identity to be inextricably linked with their childhood experiences.[15] They viewed both the victim and the survivor discourses as stigmatising and rejected these identities.[16] Those men and women telling a *narrative of normal sexual development* or *a silence recently broken* also didn't want to be seen as victims or survivors since they upheld, until relatively recently, that they had not been affected by their childhood experiences.

The other half did relate to the victim or survivor discourses. For those women telling a *narrative of the need to remember and the need to forget, protecting and helping others*, or *justice at any cost*, these discourses underpinned their thinking about their experiences and appeared to have helped them to come to terms with them. They felt a sense of solidarity with other victims or survivors.[17] These discourses can be helpful and empowering for some people and off-putting and disempowering for others. This understanding contributes to the knowledge base for clinicians working in the field and influences how we work with relational injuries.

HOW TO HEAL RELATIONAL INJURIES

To date, child protection policy and research have been balanced between the needs of the criminal justice system and the need for child protection and family support services. Much of the focus has been placed on child sexual abuse rather than on the continuum of family violence and dysfunction. However, this policy and research focus has not led to a substantial reduction in child sexual abuse. Indeed, between 1999–2000 and 2003–4 notifications in Australia doubled and substantiations increased significantly.[18] This doesn't necessarily mean that there was an increase in the number of incidents, since there have been significant changes in the mandatory reporting system for child abuse and neglect. Unfortunately, increased notifications have not led to improved outcomes for families.[19] A broader framework that positions childhood sexual experiences with adults as a social health issue is required.[20]

This book highlights the need for better provision of treatment services for adults when they make a disclosure, for men as well as for women. The nature of the treatment services to be provided is discussed in this section which covers the need for health professionals to: focus on relational injuries rather than abusive events; avoid labelling and pathologising people; frame the discussion around childhood sexual experiences not abuse; and customise their approach to gender and sexual orientation.

Focus on relational injuries rather than abusive events

The road to recovery from childhood sexual experiences with an adult can be achieved through creating healthy relationships with others. There is no need to privilege the therapeutic relationship with clinicians because other relationships are just as, if not more, valuable in this process. The focus in therapy needs to be on the relational injuries caused by these events and how they were brought about, not on the events themselves. Helping people to develop and maintain healthy, loving, life-sustaining relationships with others becomes the main priority. In terms of attachment theory this is the equivalent of developing secure adult attachment relationships, through repairing the disruption to the attachment system caused in childhood.[21]

Attachment theory predicts that people who have been sexually abused form internal working models of themselves as both victims and victimisers.[22] These internalised models affect the ways in which they behave in their relationships with other adults and leave them unable to protect themselves and, therefore, vulnerable to re-victimisation. Clinicians need to provide a secure and protective attachment relationship, in order to teach them as adults to internalise working models of how to be effective self-protectors and to contain their aggression towards others.

Perhaps the core issue is that people who have experienced relational injuries need to develop empathy, firstly for themselves as children and secondly for others. They need to begin to see themselves empathically, as a victim of circumstances beyond their control rather than as the cause of the problem. They need to recognise that the adult was in control and responsible for what happened. They then need to develop empathy for others, in order to be able to develop healthy relationships. Such an approach does not necessarily include developing a relationship with the victimiser, since forgiving others is not always possible or helpful.

It is important to recognise the danger of re-traumatisation involved in therapeutic work of this kind. Holocaust survivors have described their difficulties in creating an integrative narrative in therapy and their choice to place their traumatic experiences in a capsule separate from other aspects of their lives.[23] Clinicians need to avoid the temptation to persuade clients to confront traumatic material against their better judgement.[24] Talking about the sexual contact itself may not always be necessary or beneficial. Clients who are recovering memories may be particularly vulnerable to what could be described as self-harm sanctioned by therapy. Therapy can become a repetitive process of recovering memories and result in the re-victimisation of the client, through obliging her or him to re-experience the trauma vortex repeatedly.[25] In cases of chronic child sexual abuse, Herman wisely recommended basing therapy on a few 'paradigmatic incidents, with the understanding that one episode stands for many'.[26]

Avoid labelling or making assumptions

Some of those telling a *narrative of a silence recently broken* did not describe their experiences as abusive or traumatic for many years and those telling a *narrative of normal sexual development* remained convinced that their experiences were not abusive. This suggests that clinicians should avoid making assumptions and labelling the client's experiences in this way since such a decision is best made by the client. About half rejected the imposition of such a label on their experiences, either preferring to see them as not having impacted on them as in a *narrative of normal sexual development* or *a silence recently broken*, or as being an unhelpful and potentially stigmatising label as in the *narrative of remaining defiant*.

Many therapists advocate naming the abuse as unacceptable in situations of ongoing risk to the child,[27] and when adults recall previously unrecognised sexually abusive incidents from childhood. It is important at this point to differentiate between working with a family, in which child maltreatment is currently taking place, and working with an adult who had childhood sexual experiences with an adult many years previously. In the former situation, it is important for the clinician to confront the issue of sexual abuse with family members and to name the abuse, in order to oblige victimisers to take responsibility for their actions. However, my research suggests that adults who have had childhood sexual experiences should be allowed to come to their own conclusions about the issue of abuse, rather than have their experiences named or labelled by someone else.

Having said that, for some people there was a sense of relief when they realised that they had been the victim of a crime and were not responsible for what had happened to them. This was particularly true for those telling a *narrative of the need to remember and the need to forget, protecting and helping others* or *justice at any cost*. For them, the realisation of victimhood was often an important step in the process towards an evolving sense of themselves as able to break the cycle of abuse and hold the victimiser responsible for the crime.

Labelling all childhood sexual experiences with an adult as traumatic is not advisable, as demonstrated by those telling a *narrative of normal sexual development* or *a narrative of a silence recently broken*. Although child sexual abuse is frequently a distressing experience for a child or an adolescent and can cause symptoms of post-traumatic stress disorder, this is not inevitable in all cases. Some experiences may be less traumatic and some children may display more resilience in the face of adversity than others. It needs to be remembered that many children are asymptomatic and that less than 20% go on to experience serious psychopathology in adulthood.[28]

Frame discussion around childhood sexual experiences

A recommendation from this study is that people struggling with relational difficulties should be asked about their childhood sexual experiences, rather than about their experiences of child sexual abuse. Framing the question in this way will give those who do not view their sexual experiences with adults as abusive a forum in which to discuss them and is more likely to generate a dialogue. It is also recommended to ask both women and men about these experiences, rather than failing to ask boys or men. It is then important to provide abuse-focused treatment for men once a disclosure has been made.

When the men in this study were asked to describe their childhood sexual experiences, they were open and described the events of childhood freely. If they had been asked whether or not they had been sexually abused as children, some would have answered the question. However, those men telling a *narrative of normal sexual development* or *a narrative of a silence recently broken* would have denied this description of their experiences and would have been unlikely to describe their childhood sexual experiences. Those men telling the *narrative of remaining defiant* might have answered but would have baulked at any description that covertly placed them in the role of a victim.

Adopt a gender-sensitive approach to treatment

Gender differences in this field are of great importance and need to be taken into account more in therapy. The lack of a theoretical approach that satisfactorily explains these significant gender differences has led to a one-size-fits-all approach to service delivery for girls and boys, women and men. However, men are more reluctant than women to disclose their experiences, to have them labelled as abusive, or to be labelled themselves as victims or survivors. They are more likely than women to use avoidant coping strategies, less likely to seek help, and may experience greater relational difficulties than women. Finally, men are also more likely than women to move from victim to victimiser.

Men do not embrace therapy easily for any psychological problem, let alone for such a complex and personal issue as child sexual abuse. This creates a dilemma for clinicians, which is reinforced by the way in which therapy requires people to be emotionally open and vulnerable. Therefore, clinicians need to take into account these gender differences and actively provide gender-sensitive therapy. I believe that it is best to approach this issue tangentially with men – perhaps through a discussion of their childhood sexual experiences as discussed above. Men need to know that they will not be judged or seen as weak. The language used to describe childhood experiences needs to derive from the man himself. The adaptive value of emotional inexpressiveness for men also needs to be acknowledged, and the environment for therapy needs to be welcoming and user-friendly for men.

Most services do not recognise the need for greater provision of services for adults who make a disclosure, particularly for men. For example, in rural Australia the services operating are mainly sexual assault counselling services, which were originally set up to counsel women. Additional services designed specifically for men in rural areas need to be provided, particularly given that a history of child abuse is a better predictor of past and current suicidality than a current diagnosis of depression.[29] Telehealth technologies also need to be developed to enhance the clinical skills of rural clinicians in this field using improved consultancy arrangements.[30]

TEN-WEEK, STEP-BY-STEP RECOVERY PROGRAMME

The following is a brief guide to a 10-week, step-by-step recovery programme that I have designed for men and women who have had unwanted childhood sexual experiences which they now feel uncomfortable or distressed about. This programme is designed to be run as group therapy for men and women separately, or for people to work through individually or with the help and support of a therapist.

In this programme, men and women are invited to examine their childhood sexual experiences and decide which, if any, they remain concerned about now. They discuss what prevented them from telling anyone at the time and whether or not their fears and concerns were realistic. They explore what coping mechanisms and strategies they adopted as children in order to survive, and decide whether or not they still see these as effective. They look at ways in which they are more than the sum of their particular childhood experiences. They decide whether or not they need to tell anyone about what happened to them, plan how they would go about doing this, and consider carefully the likely repercussions for themselves and others. They examine the effect of their childhood experiences on the development of their relationships in childhood, in adolescence and in adulthood. They decide whether or not they suffered relational injuries and what needs to change now in their intimate lives and close relationships. Finally, they review all that they have learned about themselves in the programme, and decide what particular narrative to tell themselves and others about their childhood sexual experiences in future.

Week 1: My childhood sexual experiences – What happened to me back then
Week 2: Why didn't I tell anyone? – Fear, shame, blame, homosexuality
Week 3: Feeling angry and behaving badly – How I coped as a child
Week 4: It didn't affect me; I don't dwell on it – Getting on with my life
Week 5: I survived! – Overcoming adversity and protecting/helping others
Week 6: I am bigger than all this – I am more than the sum of my experiences
Week 7: Should I tell anyone now? – Telling the police, my family, my partner
Week 8: Will I become a child abuser? – Will it affect my intimate life?
Week 9: How can I create better relationships with my family and others? – Relational injury and what needs to change
Week 10: How I see myself now – What I have learned

This programme differs from other approaches in that it does not focus on the process of remembering or describing the traumatic events of childhood, or on processing traumatic memories. Neither does it focus on the symptoms of PTSD or other mental health problems, or how to overcome these. Instead it takes a strength-based approach and focuses on how people cope with childhood adversity and the narratives that they choose to tell about their experiences. It focuses on the relational injuries caused by both the childhood sexual experiences and the coping mechanisms adopted in childhood and adolescence. There is no assumption that the person views their experiences as traumatic or abusive, although some may come to this conclusion during the process. It is recommended that men and women meet in separate groups because of the significant differences between the genders in terms of responses to childhood sexual experiences.

Clearly, recovery from childhood sexual experiences does not always happen in 10 short weeks. There may be issues, such as relationship difficulties or problems related to sexual intimacy, which will take a lot longer to resolve. When a child puts their trust in an adult who destroys that trust, this can leave lasting damage to that person's ability to trust other people and to become close to them. This programme is intended as a starting point, to enable men and women to think through their childhood experiences, how they coped as children, how they are coping now, and what needs to change for them to lead more satisfying lives in future.

HOW TO SUPPORT LOVED ONES

Many of you reading this book will have had a loved one who was sexually abused as a child. Some of you will know of families who are struggling with this issue right now. You may be wondering what you can do to help them. Being there for them is the most important gift you can offer.

We know how extremely difficult it is for people, particularly men, to talk about being sexually abused as children. But unless they tell someone, no one can help them to recover from their experiences and their victimisers cannot be stopped or sanctioned in any way. The first step to recovery is normally telling someone what has happened. Of course, some people do get over their experiences without professional help, as demonstrated by some of the people that you have met in this book. They are exceptional individuals who have showed great courage and strength. However, even they told their intimate partners about their experiences.

The main reasons that people don't tell are that they are frightened of the consequences of telling, either for themselves or for other people, or they feel ashamed or to blame for what has happened to them. They are also fearful that they won't be believed and that the situation won't change for the better. In fact, it might even get worse and they might be punished for telling. This is particularly true for children, but many of these feelings linger long into adulthood.

So the most useful thing that you can do for anyone is to offer them the opportunity to tell you about their childhood sexual experiences, without the negative consequences that they fear. They need to feel free to tell you what happened to them, in as much or as little detail as they want, and how it affected them. They need you to listen without judgement, so that they don't feel any worse about it than they probably already do. It is better if you don't label what has happened to them as child sexual abuse or rape, unless they do themselves, because their experiences may have been very confusing for them and even felt loving at the time. The steps in the process are as follows.

1 Listen and allow them to talk about what happened, without labelling their experiences for them or judging their behaviour.
2 Encourage them to talk about their feelings and how they believe they have been affected by what happened to them.
3 Keep the conversation confidential, if at all possible. Don't talk to anyone else about it without their knowledge.
4 Advise them about where they could go for professional help, should they so desire.
5 Be patient and willing to be there for the long haul.

Of course, all of this is easier said than done. Often we close down these conversations because we don't know how to react. What can we say to comfort our loved one, when we are feeling so horrified by what they have been through? Can we believe what we are hearing? How do we manage our own feelings of guilt about what has happened? Do we need to make a report to authorities about an ongoing situation of child sexual abuse? How will they feel if we break their confidence? Will it feel like another betrayal? Will it automatically involve them in a court case that may be traumatic for them?

All of these are complex issues that need careful consideration. Therapists and other health professionals in many countries are obliged to make a report if the child sexual abuse is ongoing. Many will encourage people to make a self-report, even if the events happened many years ago. But as a private individual, you will need to make up your own mind about this. However, you need to be aware that if you make it clear that you will report child maltreatment, this may well limit what your loved one will feel able to tell you.

The relational injuries are the hardest things to heal, particularly when basic trust has been destroyed and when boundaries have become blurred. If you were a part of the family when these childhood events were taking place, your loved one may go through periods of feeling very angry with you for failing to protect them. This may be totally unfair, depending on the circumstances. You may have been totally unaware of what was happening. You may not have been in a position yourself to be able to protect anyone other than yourself. Be reassured that these feelings are likely to pass and that, if your loved one is willing to talk to you about them, this is a major step forward in the healing process for you both. Try to clarify your role in the situation, without becoming too defensive, since this will help others to understand their past experiences and to move forward gradually. Attending family therapy is also an option, if the situation becomes too strained between you.

Please remember that not all childhood sexual experiences are traumatic and not all victims are 'damaged goods'. Most men and women transcend their childhood experiences and go on to become contributing adults and good parents to their own children. Meeting childhood adversity head on tends to make them sensitive to the suffering of others which, while painful, can also be life-enhancing.

HOW YOUR ATTITUDES MAY HAVE CHANGED

In Chapter 1, I encouraged you to answer a questionnaire about your attitudes to child sexual abuse. I would encourage you now to go back and fill it in again, and compare your answers to determine how, if at all, your attitudes to this complex subject have changed by reading this book. My own attitudes have certainly changed since I started researching this topic.

My own personal learning

On a personal level, my own experience of loss and grief forced me to embark on a particular journey which involved building a career as a helper of others who have experienced losses of one kind or another. Conducting this research project has opened my eyes to the ways in which I have been affected by my clients,[31] and by the social construction of masculinity and femininity. Echoes of prejudice against paedophiles can be found in my own views of victimisers before starting this project. At that time I wrote 'not all victims of abuse become offenders and not all offenders are victims. Therefore these men make a conscious choice to offend. Offenders are often callous, feel no remorse, and use denial to protect themselves from guilt.' Now, having read the literature and interviewed nine men, I feel somewhat differently. I would argue that men who have damaging childhood sexual experiences with adults are constrained by the dictates of traditional masculinity not to show weakness or vulnerability or to talk about their experiences, partly for fear of being labelled as homosexual. If their relational injuries are too severe, they may go on to victimise others and some will feel great shame about their behaviour.

I am now much more open to the idea that childhood sexual experiences happen to people of both genders. I believe that I am more effective at drawing out the story of their childhood sexual experiences, particularly from men. I understand the difficulties of disclosure and how it links to so-called avoidant coping mechanisms and gender socialisation. I feel much more hopeful about people's abilities to transcend their childhood experiences and I am less likely to dwell on the experiences themselves in therapy. I am much more selective in my language in relation to this issue and will wait for my clients to name their experiences and develop their own narrative for themselves. My personal tapestry is all the richer for writing this book.

SUMMARY

Key points

- This study adds to our knowledge about childhood sexual experiences and the relational injury that can result. Relational injury is defined as a *deep wound to a close relationship*.
- Important gender differences have been highlighted, including the possibility that relational injury is more severe for boys since, often, they have fewer relational skills, are socialised not to show vulnerability or weakness, and are less likely to disclose what has happened or to seek help.
- There are significant developmental difficulties in disclosure for children of both sexes and for adults. Preconditions for disclosure are rarely found within dysfunctional families.
- There is a wide range of resilient narratives that men and women can tell about their childhood sexual experiences, in order to explain them to themselves and to others. These include, but are not limited to, the current socially acceptable 'victim' and 'survivor' narratives which are sometimes viewed as stigmatising since they link the person's identity to their childhood experiences so directly.
- These findings have implications for health professionals. They suggest that it would be advantageous to focus on the relational injury caused by childhood events, and not on the abusive events themselves.
- It is important not to label someone else's childhood sexual experiences as traumatic or abusive, or to define them as a victim or a survivor, unless they do so themselves.
- It is sensible to frame the discussion around childhood sexual experiences, rather than child sexual abuse, at least to begin with. This will make it easier for people, and men in particular, to be more open about their lives.
- It is important to adopt a gender-sensitive approach to this work and to recognise the significance of gender socialisation in relation to this issue.
- A 10-week, step-by-step programme is described for working with groups of men or women.
- Suggestions for supporting loved ones are made including listening without labelling or judging, encouraging them to talk about their feelings and the impact, keeping the conversation confidential, giving advice about seeking professional help and being patient.

For this book, a wide variety of people were interviewed about their childhood sexual experiences. For many, but not all, these experiences were damaging to their early relationships with family members. Some were still coming to terms with their experiences and described their ongoing suffering. Most managed to tell positive and resilient narratives to others, despite their experiences. Many women had been transformed by their experiences, often through relational means, and saw themselves as protecting and helping others or as seeking justice for future generations. Some people had remained defiant and refused to be defined by their childhood sexual experiences. Some claimed not to have been affected by their experiences, although they were beginning to be concerned about the impact on their ability to create and maintain intimate relationships with others.

People chose to be interviewed because they hoped that, by coming forward and telling their stories, they might be able to help other people – either by preventing children from being harmed or by helping adults to come to terms with their own childhood experiences. I, too, hope that you will be affected by these stories of stoicism, protectiveness, bravery and defiance, and will continue to work towards the eradication of child maltreatment in our society.

Ten-week, step-by-step recovery programme

The following is a brief guide to a 10-week, step-by-step recovery programme that I have designed for adults who had unwanted childhood sexual experiences which they now feel uncomfortable or distressed about in some way. I would encourage you to work through these steps with a therapist rather than on your own. You might find it useful to write a journal during the process.

WEEK 1: MY CHILDHOOD SEXUAL EXPERIENCES – WHAT HAPPENED TO ME BACK THEN

Take an honest inventory of your childhood and the family environment in which you grew up. Focus on any experiences which could now be seen as abusive, physically, sexually, emotionally or spiritually. Think about your experiences within the home environment, at school, at church, with other children, with other adults and so on. Decide which, if any, of your childhood sexual experiences would nowadays be seen as abusive and which, if any, are you still worried about. These will become the focus for recovery.

Exercise 1: Burn or otherwise destroy your list of childhood experiences that no longer concern you and try to forgive all those people who were involved in some way, either actively or passively. If you find yourself unable to forgive someone, perhaps you need to add this particular childhood experience to your list of those that still concern you in some way.

WEEK 2: WHY DIDN'T I TELL ANYONE? – FEAR, SHAME, BLAME, HOMOSEXUALITY

You probably haven't told anyone what happened to you as a child. Of course, there are many good reasons why children don't tell. You may have been fearful of the consequences for yourself or for other family members. You may have felt ashamed about what happened to you or blamed yourself and taken responsibility for what happened, especially if you were an adolescent at the time. It may have been particularly hard for you because your experiences were homosexual in nature. Try to work out how realistic your feelings were at the time, given your particular family context. And work out how frightened and ashamed you feel now. Do you still blame yourself for what happened?

Exercise 2: Think about your childhood sexual experiences that still concern you. Write down a brief description of what happened and how you felt about it at the time. If you had decided to tell someone at the time, what would have been the likely consequences for you, your siblings, and other family members? Decide whether or not you made the right decision not to tell anyone back then. Also decide whether or not your feelings of fear, shame or self-blame are still appropriate and helpful to you.

WEEK 3: FEELING ANGRY AND BEHAVING BADLY – HOW I COPED AS A CHILD

Think about how you behaved as an adolescent and young adult. Some of your behaviour may have been as a result of childhood sexual experiences. You may have felt angry and betrayed and shown it by behaving in a violent way, by using drugs or alcohol to escape from painful feelings or by becoming involved in non-committed sex or abusive relationships. Alternatively, you may have withdrawn into a shell and refused to have close relationships with other people. While many of these behaviours can be understood as a response to childhood sexual experiences, they are not necessarily excusable.

Exercise 3: Take an inventory of your poor behaviour in adolescence and young adulthood. Who was it aimed at? Was it effective? Who did it hurt the most? Make a list of anyone who deserves an apology from you now. Write down a creative way in which you would like to make amends to each of these people, without necessarily explaining anything to them. Carry these actions out, if you wish.

WEEK 4: IT DIDN'T AFFECT ME, I DON'T DWELL ON IT – GETTING ON WITH MY LIFE

Many people, especially men, believe that their childhood sexual experiences did not affect them badly. They have been able to lead satisfying lives in adulthood. Decide what impact, if any, your experiences have had on your life. Were your childhood sexual experiences a normal part of your sexual development? Were you able to put them to one side and move on with your life? Did you find it relatively easy not to think about what had happened? Was there someone or some event that helped you to put it all behind them? What strategies did you use in childhood to avoid thinking about these experiences? Were these useful, creative and functional ways of demonstrating resilience or have they caused you further harm?

Exercise 4: Imagine that you have put all your thoughts and feelings about your child-hood sexual experiences in a box or suitcase. Take it out and examine your thoughts and feelings carefully, including the ones you identified in week 2. Decide which ones should stay where they were, and which ones need to change. Put some back in the box or suitcase and put it away. Monitor any changes in the other thoughts and feelings that occur as you work your way through this 10-week programme.

WEEK 5: I SURVIVED! – OVERCOMING ADVERSITY AND PROTECTING/HELPING OTHERS

If you are continuing with this programme, your childhood sexual experiences are obviously bothering you. Perhaps they involved an abuse of trust. Perhaps you were sensible not to talk about them at the time, given your family situation and your lack of support at the time. You may have been able to make a positive life for yourself. Read the stories of how other people have coped. By understanding how other people have been able to overcome similar childhood experiences and create a positive narrative about themselves as protecting or helping others or as seeking justice, you will be able to formulate a more positive view of your own responses to events.

Exercise 5: You have heard about how other people have coped with childhood sexual experiences. Having heard so many different stories, which one resonates the most with you? How do you see your response to your childhood experiences now? Did you need to protect yourself? Did you try to protect others? Did you get angry? Did you try to tell anyone? Now imagine a child that you know who is the same age as you were when these events happened. What do you think that child would have been able to do in the same circumstances? Accept that you were a child, and that you behaved like a child, and that you did the best that you could do at the time. Light a candle or say a prayer or read a poem for you as a child.

WEEK 6: I AM BIGGER THAN ALL THIS – I AM MORE THAN THE SUM OF MY EXPERIENCES

Focus on who you are beyond your childhood sexual experiences. Although these experiences may have had a lasting impact, they do not make up the whole of you. Read the stories of how other people have transcended their childhood sexual experiences and do not necessarily want their identities to be tied to this one aspect of their lives. They describe their spiritual growth, their desire to help others and their rejection of the potentially stigmatising label of being a victim or a survivor of child sexual abuse.

Exercise 6: See yourself as a whole person. Describe who you are and what defines you. Write a brief description, using five adjectives that capture the essence of who you are. Ask your friends and family to describe who they think that you are. Draw a timeline and put on it every significant event that has happened to you. Put your early sexual experiences into context as a part, but not the whole of you.

WEEK 7: SHOULD I TELL ANYONE NOW? – TELLING THE POLICE, MY FAMILY, MY PARTNER

The question of whether or not you should tell anyone now, as an adult, is an important one to consider. Think hard about who you want to tell and what your motives are. Think through this issue very carefully because making a disclosure may have some serious consequences, not just for you but for other family members. You also need to consider the consequences of not telling before taking any action.

Exercise 7: Decide who it is that you want to tell. Work out what your real motives are. Think through the likely consequences of telling. Try to be realistic about it. If possible, check out your ideas with someone that you trust before putting them into practice. Remember that the consequences can be unexpected, because people prefer to remain ignorant about such experiences and often do not want to know about them. Only decide to tell someone if you believe that the negative consequences are worth it, or if you feel compelled to do so in some way and have thought through the consequences of telling and not telling.

WEEK 8: WILL I BECOME A CHILD ABUSER? – WILL IT AFFECT MY INTIMATE LIFE?

This is an important question that many people who have had childhood sexual experiences with adults ask themselves at some time. Most people do not go on to become abusive themselves. Think about the impact of these experiences on your sex life and your intimate relationships with others.

Exercise 8: Be honest with yourself about your sexual desires. Do they include an attraction towards children? Are you concerned that you might act on these desires in any way? If so, you need to go and talk to a health professional about this issue.

WEEK 9: HOW CAN I CREATE BETTER RELATIONSHIPS WITH MY FAMILY AND OTHERS? – RELATIONAL INJURY AND WHAT NEEDS TO CHANGE

When someone has kept a secret for a long time, this tends to affect their relationships with other people. Look at the relationships within your family, using a diagram or a family tree, and decide which relationships have been negatively affected by your childhood sexual experiences. What is the problem in the relationship? Is it a lack of trust, an inability to be honest and open with each other, or perhaps feelings of anger that constantly surface? These problems have taken years to develop and will not be resolved in a 10-week course. But try to identify issues with family members that need to be resolved in the future and gradually work towards that.

Exercise 9: *Draw your family tree. Join people with coloured lines to represent the relationships that you have with them now (e.g. close relationship, too close and over-involved, angry and constantly fighting, never speak to one another, distant and uninvolved etc.). Decide which, if any, of these relationships have been damaged by the events of your childhood, and which need to be repaired. Think about some ways that you might gradually repair them.*

WEEK 10: HOW I SEE MYSELF NOW – WHAT I HAVE LEARNED

Review everything that you have learned as a result of working through the programme. Summarise your story using a new narrative of resilience that you intend to tell about their experiences from now on. Make a commitment to make certain changes in your life and your relationships in the future.

Exercise 10: *Write up your response to this programme and consider posting it on a blog site for others to read. This may help them in ways you cannot imagine.*

Research methodology

Narrative inquiry methodology was used in this study. Participants were recruited through the use of advertising in local newspapers and on local radio. As a result, a purposive sample of participants was recruited.[1] All those interviewed were interested in being involved in a study of early sexual experiences. In order to be eligible to participate in the study people had to:

➤ be aged between 25 and 70 years old
➤ have had a sexual experience at the age of 15 or under with an adult
➤ not be currently under the care of a psychiatrist.

The term *early sexual experience* was not specifically defined, allowing the participants the freedom to interpret the term in any way they wished. In order to avoid recruiting participants into the study who were currently suffering from a mental illness and, therefore, more likely to be emotionally vulnerable, participants were excluded if they were currently under the care of a psychiatrist. Participants older than 70 were also excluded from the sample in order to limit the time period involved in the study.

A convenience sample was recruited through local press and radio. In this process, care was taken not to describe early sexual experiences as abusive, although the participants themselves often did so during the interview process. Following each burst of advertising, a number of potential participants contacted me by phone or e-mail. Before conducting an interview I checked that the potential participants fulfilled the requirements for the study.

It was important to interview both men and women since gender was an important discriminator in this field. Indeed whether or not the experiences were homosexual or heterosexual was also important, but it was decided not to recruit on this basis, given the sensitivity of the questions that would need to be asked in order to establish this at such an early stage of the process.

Details of participants recruited

Table 1 shows a breakdown of participants in terms of their sex, age, sexual orientation, the nature of their early sexual experiences and the extent to which they have attended therapy in the past. There were 13 women interviewed and nine men, making a total sample of 22. Twenty of the 22 participants who volunteered for the study identified as heterosexual. The women who volunteered were younger than the men on average and were more likely to have had heterosexual, incestuous early sexual experiences with their fathers or stepfathers. The women interviewed were also more likely than the men to have attended therapy, often for 10 or more sessions.

TABLE 1 Characteristics of participants by gender

	Total	*Female*	*Male*
Age			
25–35	4	3	1
36–45	7	7	0
46–55	9	3	6
55–70	2	0	2
Sexual orientation			
Heterosexual	20	12	8
Homosexual/Lesbian/Bisexual	2	1	1
Adult involved in ESE			
Father, stepfather or relative	11	10	1
Other male	7	3	4
Adults of both sexes	3	0	3
Other female	1	0	1
Nature of ESE			
Heterosexual experiences	14	13	1
Homosexual experiences	5	0	5
Heterosexual and homosexual	3	0	3
Therapy attended			
None	6	2	4
1–10 sessions	4	2	2
10+ sessions	12	9	3
Total	22	13	9

All of the men who volunteered for the study, bar one, were over 45 years old. Five of the nine men had experienced physical, sexual and emotional abuse in the homes that they had grown up in, not necessarily with their biological parents. Most had either homosexual experiences with men that were known to them or with adults of both sexes. Four had never attended therapy sessions. It should be noted that no women volunteered to take part in the study who had been sexually abused by another woman. Perhaps being victimised by a woman remains even more taboo in our society.[2]

Participants came from all walks of life. Twelve participants had received a university education, five had completed vocational training, and five had had little tertiary education. Four worked in the helping professions, three were teachers, three were engineers, one was a technician and one was self-employed. Three identified their occupation as being a mother and two as full-time carers. Two were on pensions, two were unemployed, and one was currently working as a truck driver. Sixteen identified their ethnic origin as Australian, two as New Zealanders and four as having Australian/European backgrounds.

The interview context

At the start of the interview I read through the information sheet with the participant. I explained that I would remove all identifying details from their stories in order to protect their confidentiality. I also explained that I would give each participant a pseudonym so that other people reading the book would not be able to identify them. A few participants chose their own, often symbolic, pseudonyms and others wanted to use their real names but I decided to over-rule their wishes and allocated them a pseudonym later. This was done after consultation with my PhD supervisors in the belief that participants could not necessarily predict how their stories might be quoted and in what contexts they might be retold.

I explained the limits of confidentiality to participants, by stating that in the event that I was told that a child was being sexually or physically abused, I would be obliged to inform the New South Wales Department of Community Services. This information was also included on the consent form that all participants were asked to sign before the interview began.

I also reassured participants that they had the right to terminate the interview at any time if they wished to do so. This was because of the ethical concern that the interview process could be potentially re-traumatising to participants. However, no participants chose to terminate the interview early. I also reassured them that if they changed their minds about participating in the study during or after the interview process, I would erase the tape recording and not use the information collected in any way. No one asked me to do so. I also encouraged participants to stop the interview whenever they felt they needed a break. This often happened quite naturally when the tape recorder clicked off after

45 minutes. I always enquired whether or not the participant would like to take a break or would like to stop at that point. This offer was accepted by some participants. Finally, I told participants that I would be able to provide referrals to local counselling agencies if they became upset during the interview.

Limitations of the research methodology

All qualitative research methodologies have a similar limitation in relation to quantitative methodologies, in that the data is collected from a relatively small number of people who are not necessarily representative of a particular population. The narrative inquiry methodology used had four additional limitations.

1 The people were recruited through the media and were 'volunteers'.
2 The findings did not represent the 'truth' but a reconstruction of events.
3 The findings were limited to a particular historical, social and cultural reference point.
4 My behaviour inevitably influenced the narratives that were told.

These limitations will be discussed in turn.

As a qualitative study the project was intended to be exploratory in nature. It would have been impossible to determine what would comprise a representative sample of people who have had childhood sexual experiences, at the age of 15 or under with someone over the age of 18. Indeed the definition of what constitutes an 'early' sexual experience would differ from culture to culture and even between states. Most of the available data relates to the prevalence of child sexual abuse, rather than to childhood sexual experiences. Research based on samples of survivors of child sexual abuse omit a large proportion of people who have technically been sexually abused as children, but who do not experience the sexual contact as abusive or do not chose, for whatever reason, to define themselves as victims or survivors of child sexual abuse.

In practice, this qualitative research project was based on a convenience sample of people who volunteered to be interviewed about their childhood sexual experiences. Inevitably, this did leave gaps within the sample. For example, no women volunteered to be interviewed who had childhood sexual experiences with women. Similarly, no men volunteered who had childhood sexual experiences with their fathers or stepfathers.

It might be assumed that these volunteers might perhaps be somewhat exhibitionist in nature, or even have fabricated their stories in order to gain attention. Of course, it is impossible to know the veracity of the stories told. However, I agree with Dorais who stated 'I have never received that impression [exhibitionist] from the people I have interviewed. On the contrary, in many cases, I was one of the first in whom they confided.'[1] People willingly volunteered because they wanted to help others. They found the interview a useful and satisfying experience, which helped them to realise how far they had already travelled in terms of overcoming their childhood experiences and, in some cases, to recognise the road still left to travel.

The study did not set out to find out the 'truth' about childhood sexual experiences and the findings were based on the reconstruction of memories of events that took place at least a decade before. People reconstructed the events of childhood, in a topic area for which memories have been scrutinised and found to be unreliable. Given the social construction of these narratives, this represented the 'narrative truth' for these particular people.[2]

The findings were limited to a particular historical, social and cultural reference point. Those interviewed all lived in cities, small towns or rural areas of New South Wales, Australia. A few were from European migrant backgrounds but none was from Asian migrant backgrounds, first-generation migrants or Indigenous Australians. Hence the sample was limited to adult members of mainstream Australian society. All of the childhood sexual experiences described had taken place between the 1950s and the 1990s but were being examined from the perspective of Australians living in the post-millennium period. How similar these experiences are to those of people living in Los Angeles, Jerusalem, Bangkok or rural areas of Nepal is for the reader to decide.

Suggested reading and websites

Briere J, Scott C. *Principles of Trauma Therapy: a guide to symptoms, evaluation, and treatment.* Thousand Oaks, California: Sage Publications; 2006.

Briggs F. *From Victim to Offender: how child sexual abuse victims become offenders.* St Leonard's, Australia: Allen & Unwin; 1995.

Cameron C. *Resolving Childhood Trauma: a long-term study of abuse survivors.* Thousand Oaks, California: Sage Publications; 2000.

Darlington Y. *Moving On: women's experiences of childhood sexual abuse and beyond.* Sydney, Australia: The Federation Press; 1996.

Dorais M. *Don't Tell: the sexual abuse of boys.* Quebec: McGill-Queens; 2002.

Draucker CB, Martsolf DS. *Counselling Survivors of Childhood Sexual Abuse.* 3rd ed. London: Sage Publications; 2006.

Durham A. *Young Men Surviving Child Sexual Abuse: research stories and lessons for therapeutic practice.* London: NSPCC/Wiley; 2003.

Faller KC. *Interviewing Children about Sexual Abuse: controversies and best practice.* Oxford: Oxford University Press; 2007.

Finkelhor D. *Child Sexual Abuse: new theory and research.* New York: The Free Press; 1984.

Friedrich WN. *Psychological Assessment of Sexually Abused Children and Their Families.* Thousand Oaks, California: Sage Publications; 2002.

Herman JL. *Trauma and Recovery: from domestic abuse to political terror.* Hammersmith, London: Pandora; 1994.

Jenkins P. *Moral Panic: changing concepts of the child molester in modern America.* New Haven: Yale University Press; 1998.

Richardson S, Bacon H, editors. *Creative Responses to Child Sexual Abuse: challenges and dilemmas.* London: Jessica Kingsley; 2001.

Sanderson C. *Counselling Adult Survivors of Child Sexual Abuse.* 3rd ed. London: Jessica Kingsley; 2006.

Warner S. *Understanding Child Sexual Abuse: making the tactics visible.* Gloucester: Handsell Publishing; 2000.

Australian Centre for Child Protection www.unisa.edu.au/childprotection/

Australian Federal Police www.afp.gov.au

Australian Institute of Criminology www.aic.gov.au

Australian Institute of Family Studies www.aifs.gov.au/

Australian Institute of Health and Welfare www.aihw.gov.au/

Beyond Blue – Australian National Depression Initiative www.beyondblue.org.au/

Coorey Report on Child Sexual Abuse in Rural and Remote Australian Indigenous Communities www.aph.gov.au/SENATE/committee/indigenousaffairs_ctte/

Health Insite – Australian Government Initiative www.healthinsite.gov.au/

Kids Helpline www.kidshelp.com.au/

NAPCAN National Association for Preventing Child Abuse and Neglect www.napcan.org.au/

References

Chapter 1 Childhood sexual experiences

1 May-Chahal C, Cawson P. Measuring child maltreatment in the United Kingdom: a study of the prevalence of child abuse and neglect. *Child Abuse Negl.* 2005; **29**: 969–84.

2 Warner S. Disrupting identity through Visible Therapy. In: Reavey P, Warner S, editors. *New Feminist Studies of Child Sexual Abuse: sexual scripts and dangerous dialogues.* London: Routledge; 2003. pp. 226–47.

3 Stanley JL, Bartholomew K, Oram D. Gay and bisexual men's age-discrepant childhood sexual experiences. *J Sex Res.* 2004; **41**(4): 381–9. Putnam FW. Ten-year research update review: child sexual abuse. *J Am Acad Child Adolesc Psychiatry.* 2003; **42**(3): 269–78.

4 Fox KV. Silent voices: a subversive reading of child sexual abuse. In: Gergen M, Gergen KJ, editors. *Social Constructionism: a reader.* London: Sage Publications; 2003. pp. 92–101.

5 Rind B, Tromovitch P, Bausermen R. A meta-analysis of assumed properties of child sexual abuse using college samples. *Psychol Bull.* 1998; **124**(1): 22–53.

6 Finkelhor D, Berliner L. Research on the treatment of sexually abused children: a review and recommendations. *J Am Acad Child Adolesc Psychiatry.* 1995; **34**(11): 1408–23. Faller KC. *Understanding and Assessing Child Sexual Maltreatment.* 2nd ed. Thousand Oaks, California: Sage Publications; 2003.

7 Herman JL. *Trauma and Recovery: from domestic abuse to political terror.* Hammersmith: Pandora; 1994.

8 Hart B. Re-authoring the stories we work by situating the narrative approach in the presence of the family of therapists. *Aust New Zeal J Fam Ther.* 1995; **16**(4): 181–9.

9 Rind B, Tromovitch P. A meta-analytic review of findings from national samples on psychological correlates of child sexual abuse. *J Sex Res.* 1997; **34**(3): 237–55. Freud S, Breuer J. *Studies on Hysteria.* London: The Hogarth Press; 1895.

10 Crossley ML. *Introducing Narrative Psychology: self, trauma and the construction of meaning.* Buckingham: Open University Press; 2000. Herman JL. Crime and memory. In: Strozier CB, Flynn M, editors. *Trauma and Self.* Maryland: Rowman & Littlefield; 1996. pp. 3–17.

11 Masten AS, Reed M-GJ. Resilience in development. In: Snyder CR, Lopez SJ, editors. *Handbook of Positive Psychology*. Oxford: Oxford University Press; 2005. pp. 74–88.

12 McNally RJ, Perlman CA, Ristuccia CS, *et al*. Clinical characteristics of adults reporting repressed, recovered, or continuous memories of childhood sexual abuse. *J Consult Clin Psychol*. 2006; **74**(2): 237–42.

13 Ibid. p. 237.

14 Bonanno GA. Loss, trauma, and human resilience: have we underestimated the human capacity to thrive after extremely aversive events? *Am Psychol*. 2004; **59**(1): 20–8. Phillips A, Daniluk JC. Beyond 'survivor': how childhood sexual abuse informs the identity of adult women at the end of the therapeutic process. *J Couns Dev*. 2004; **82**(2): 177–84.

15 Faller KC, op. cit.

16 Finkelhor D, Hotaling GT, Yllo K. *Stopping Family Violence: research priorities for the coming decade*. Newbury Park, California: Sage Publications; 1988. p. 64.

17 Rogers WS, Rogers RS. Taking the child abuse debate apart. In: Rogers WS, Hevey D, Ash E, editors. *Child Abuse and Neglect: facing the challenge*. London: The Open University; 1989. pp. 50–63.

Chapter 2 Damaged goods?

1 Hunter SV. Understanding the complexity of child sexual abuse: a review of the literature with implications for family counselling. *The Family Journal*. 2006; **14**(4): 349–58. Hunter SV. Child maltreatment in remote Aboriginal communities and the Northern Territory Emergency Response: a complex issue. *Aust Soc Work*. 2008; **61**(4): 372–88.

2 Sanderson C. *Counselling Adult Survivors of Child Sexual Abuse*. 3rd ed. London: Jessica Kingsley; 2006. p. 68.

3 May-Chahal C, Cawson P, op. cit.

4 de Visser RO, Smith AMA, Rissel CE, *et al*. Experiences of sexual coercion among a representative sample of adults. *Aust N Z J Public Health*. 2003; **27**(2): 198–203. Richters J, Rissel C. *Doing it Down Under*. St Leonard's, Australia: Allen & Unwin; 2005.

5 King MB, Coxell A, Mezey GC. The prevalence and characteristics of male sexual assault. In: Mezey GC, King MB, editors. *Male Victims of Sexual Assault*. 2nd ed. Oxford: Oxford University Press; 2000. pp. 1–15.

6 deYoung M. The world according to NAMBLA: accounting for deviance. In: Hensley C, Tewksbury R, editors. *Sexual Deviance: a reader*. Boulder, Colorado: Lynne Rienner Publishers; 2003. pp. 105–18.

7 Spataro J, Mullen PE, Burgess PM, *et al*. Impact of child sexual abuse on mental health: prospective study in males and females. *Br J Psychiatry*. 2004; **184**: 416–21.

8 Finkelhor D, Berliner L, op. cit.

9 Featherstone B. Issues of gender. In: Wilson K, James A, editors. *The Child Protection Handbook*. 3rd ed. Edinburgh: Elsevier; 2007. pp. 119–33.

10 James M. Child abuse and neglect: Part 1 – redefining the issues. *Trends and Issues in Crime and Criminal Justice*, Australian Institute of Criminology. 2000; **146**: 1–6.

11 Coid J, Petruckevitch A, Feder G, *et al*. Relation between childhood sexual and

physical abuse and risk of revictimisation in women: a cross-sectional survey. *Lancet.* 2001; **358**(9280): 450–4.

12 Sperry DM, Gilbert BO. Child peer sexual abuse: preliminary data on outcomes and disclosure experiences. *Child Abuse Negl.* 2005; **29**: 889–904.

13 Rind B, Tromovitch P, Bausermen R, op. cit.

14 Putnam FW, op. cit.

15 Gladstone GL, Parker GB, Mitchell PB, *et al.* Implications of childhood trauma for depressed women: an analysis of pathways from childhood sexual abuse to deliber- ate self-harm and revictimisation. *Am J Psychiatry.* 2004; **161**(8): 1417–25.

16 NSW Government. *Interagency Guidelines of Child Protection Intervention.* 2006 [cited 6 December 2006]. Available from: www.community.nsw.gov.au

17 Brown T, Sheehan R, Frederico M, *et al.* Child abuse in the context of parental separa- tion and divorce. *Children Australia.* 2002; **27**(2): 35–40.

18 US Department of Health and Human Services. *Child Maltreatment 2003.* Washington DC: Government Printing Office; 2005.

19 Sidebotham P, Heron J. Child maltreatment in the 'children of the nineties': a cohort study of risk factors. *Child Abuse Negl.* 2006; **30**: 497–522.

20 Australian Institute of Health and Welfare. *A Picture of Australia's Children.* Canberra: Australian Institute of Health and Welfare; 2005.

21 Jones C, Zhong X, Dempsey K, *et al. The Health and Wellbeing of Northern Territory Women: from the desert to the sea 2005.* Darwin: Department of Health and Community Services; 2005.

22 Hunter SV. Child maltreatment in remote Aboriginal communities, op. cit.

23 Findholt N, Robrecht LC. Legal and ethical considerations in research with sexually active adolescents: the requirement to report statutory rape (Comment). *Perspect Sex Reprod Health.* 2002; **34**(5): 259–64.

24 US Department of Health and Human Services, op. cit. Elliott K, Urquza A. Ethnicity, culture, and child maltreatment. *J Soc Issues.* 2006; **62**(4): 787–809.

25 Elliott K, Urquza A, op. cit.

26 Foster A. Reframing public discourse on child abuse in Australia. *Child Abuse Prevention Newsletter,* Australian Institute of Family Studies. 2005; **13**(1): 22–6.

27 Ford D. Aboriginal child sexual abuse and support services. In: Dudgeon P, Garrey D, Pickett H, editors. *Working with Indigenous Australians: a handbook for psychologists.* Perth: Gurada Press; 2000. pp. 451–6.

28 Human Rights and Equal Opportunities Commission. *Bringing Them Home: Report of the National Inquiry into the Separation of Aboriginal and Torres Strait Islander Children from their Families (Australia).* Canberra: HREOC; 1997. Bird C, editor. *The Stolen Children: their stories including extracts from the Report of the National Inquiry into the Separation of Aboriginal and Torres Strait Islander children from their families.* Milson's Point, Australia: Random House; 1998.

29 Korbin JE. Culture and child maltreatment: cultural competence and beyond. *Child Abuse Negl.* 2002; **26**: 637–44.

30 Ibid.

31 Libesman T. Indigenising Indigenous child welfare. *Indigenous Law Bulletin.* 2007; **6**(24): 17–19.

Chapter 3 Normal sexual development

1 Faller KC, op. cit.
2 Rutter M, Giller H, Hagell A. *Antisocial Behaviour in Young People*. Cambridge: Cambridge University Press; 1998. p. 170.
3 Masten AS. Ordinary magic: resilience processes in development. *Am Psychol*. 2001; **56**(3): 227–38.
4 Serbin LA, Karp J. The intergenerational transfer of psychological risk: mediators of vulnerability and resilience. *Annu Rev Psychol*. 2004; **55**: 333–63.
5 Werner EE. Resilience research: past, present, and future. In: Peters RDV, Leadbeater B, McMahon RJ, editors. *Resilience in Children, Families, and Communities*. New York: Plenum Publishers; 2005. pp. 3–11.
6 Wright MOD, Fopma-Lay J, Fischer S. Multidimensional assessment of resilience in mothers who are child sexual abuse survivors. *Child Abuse Negl*. 2005; **29**: 1173–93.
7 Dolezal C, Carballo-Dieguez A. Childhood sexual experiences and the perception of abuse among Latino men who have sex with men. *J Sex Res*. 2002; **39**(3): 165–73.
8 Stanley JL, Bartholomew K, Oram D, op. cit.
9 Freud S, Breuer J, op. cit.
10 Finkelhor D, Hotaling GT, Yllo K, op. cit. p. 64.
11 Jenkins P. *Moral Panic: changing concepts of the child molester in modern America*. New Haven: Yale University Press; 1998.

Chapter 4 A silence recently broken

1 Leitenberg, *et al*. 1992, cited in Spaccarelli S. Stress, appraisal, and coping in child sexual abuse: a theoretical and empirical review. *Psychol Bull*. 1994; **116**(2): 340–62.
2 Spaccarelli S, op. cit.
3 Himelein MJ, McElrath JAV. Resilient child sexual abuse survivors: cognitive coping and illusion. *Child Abuse Negl*. 1996; **20**(8): 747–58.
4 Darlington Y. Escape as a response to childhood sexual abuse. *J Child Sex Abus*. 1996; **5**(3): 77–93.
5 Denov MS. The long-term effects of child sexual abuse by female perpetrators: a qualitative study of male and female victims. *J Interpers Violence*. 2004; **19**(10): 1137–56. Turton J. *Child Abuse, Gender and Society*. New York: Routledge; 2008.
6 Shaw JA, Lewis JE, Loeb A, *et al*. A comparison of Hispanic and African-American sexually abused girls and their families. *Child Abuse Negl*. 2001; **25**: 1363–79.
7 Haaken J, Lamb S. The politics of child sexual abuse research. *Society*. 2000; **37**(4): 7–14.
8 Holmes GR, Offen L, Waller G. See no evil, hear no evil, speak no evil: why do relatively few male victims of childhood sexual abuse receive help for abuse-related issues in adulthood? *Clin Psychol Rev*. 1997; **17**(1): 69–88.
9 Rencken RH. *Brief and Extended Interventions in Sexual Abuse*. Alexandria: American Counseling Association; 2000.
10 Agar K, Read J. What happens when people disclose sexual or physical abuse to staff at a community health centre? *Int J Ment Health Nurs*. 2002; **11**: 70–9.
11 Banyard VL, Williams LM, Siegel JA. Childhood sexual abuse: a gender perspective on context and consequences. *Child Maltreat*. 2004; **9**(3): 223–38.

12 Lew M. *Victims No Longer: the classic guide for men recovering from sexual child abuse.* 2nd ed. New York: Harper Collins; 2004.

13 Sigmon ST, Greene MP, Rohan KJ, *et al.* Coping and adjustment in male and female survivors of childhood sexual abuse. *J Child Sex Abus.* 1996; **5**(3): 57–75. Kaplow JB, Dodge KA, Amaya-Jackson L, *et al.* Pathways to PTSD, Part II: sexually abused children. *Am J Psychiatry.* 2005; **162**(7): 1305–10.

14 London K, Bruck M, Ceci SJ, *et al.* Disclosure of child sexual abuse: what does the research tell us about ways that children tell? *Psychol Public Policy Law.* 2005; **11**(1): 194–226.

15 Kogan SM. Disclosing unwanted sexual experiences: results from a national sample of adolescent women. *Child Abuse Negl.* 2004; **28**: 147–65.

16 Dorais M. *Don't Tell: the sexual abuse of boys.* Quebec: McGill-Queens; 2002. pp. 18–19.

17 Gill M, Tutty LM. Male survivors of childhood sexual abuse: a qualitative study and issues for clinical consideration. *J Child Sex Abus.* 1999; **7**(3): 19–33.

18 Watkins B, Bentovim A. Male children and adolescents as victims: a review of current knowledge. In: Mezey GC, King MB, editors. *Male Victims of Sexual Assault.* 2nd ed. Oxford: Oxford University Press; 2000. pp. 35–77.

19 Salter D, McMillan D, Richards M, *et al.* Development of sexually abusive behaviour in sexually victimised males: a longitudinal study (Articles). *Lancet.* 2003; **361**(9356): 471–6.

Chapter 5 The need to remember and the need to forget

1 Somer E, Szwarcberg S. Variables in delayed disclosure of childhood sexual abuse. *Am J Orthopsychiatry.* 2001; **71**(3): 332.

2 Phillips A, Daniluk JC, op. cit.

3 Gilligan C. *In a Different Voice: psychological theory and woman's development.* Cambridge: Harvard University Press; 1982.

4 Fine M. Sexuality, schooling, and adolescent females: the missing discourse of desire. *Harv Educ Rev.* 1988; **58**: 29–53.

5 Welldon EV. *Mother, Madonna, Whore: the idealization and denigration of motherhood.* New York: The Guilford Press; 1988.

Chapter 6 Protecting and helping others

1 Herman JL. *Father–Daughter Incest.* Cambridge: Harvard University Press; 1981.

2 Dorias M, op. cit. Kia-Keating M, Grossman FK, Sorsoli L, *et al.* Containing and resisting masculinity: narratives of renegotiation among resilient male survivors of childhood sexual abuse. *Psychology of Men & Masculinity.* 2005; **6**(3): 169–85.

3 Courtois CA. *Healing the Incest Wound: adult survivors in therapy.* New York: WW Norton & Company; 1988.

4 Cameron C. *Resolving Childhood Trauma: a long-term study of abuse survivors.* Thousand Oaks, California: Sage Publications; 2000. p. 140.

5 Casement P. Objective fact and psychological truth: some thoughts on 'recovered memory'. In: Sinason V, editor. *Memory in Dispute.* London: Karnac Books; 1998. pp. 179–84.

6 Haaken J, Lamb S, op. cit.

Chapter 7 Justice at any cost

1 Warner S, op. cit.

2 Berliner L, Conte JR. The process of victimisation: the victims' perspective. *Child Abuse Negl.* 1990; **14**: 29–40.

3 Finkelhor D. The trauma of child sexual abuse. In: Wyatt GE, Powell GJ, editors. *Lasting Effects of Child Sexual Abuse.* Newbury Park, California: Sage Publications; 1988. pp. 61–82.

4 Spaccarelli S, op. cit.

5 Werner EE, op. cit.

6 Ullman SE, Filipas HH. Gender differences in social relations to abuse disclosures, post-abuse coping, and PTSD of child sexual survivors. *Child Abuse Negl.* 2005; **29**: 767–82.

7 Briere J, Scott C. *Principles of Trauma Therapy: a guide to symptoms, evaluation, and treatment.* Thousand Oaks, California: Sage Publications; 2006.

8 Jonzon E, Lindblad F. Risk factors and protective factors in relation to subjective health among adult female victims of child sexual abuse. *Child Abuse Negl.* 2006; **30**: 127–43.

9 Werner EE, op. cit.

Chapter 8 Remaining defiant

1 Lev-Wiesel R. Quality of life in adult survivors of childhood sexual abuse who have undergone therapy. *J Child Sex Abus.* 2000; **9**(1): 1–13.

2 Mossige S, Jensen TK, Gulbrandsen W, *et al.* Children's narratives of sexual abuse. *Narrative Inquiry.* 2005; **15**(2): 377–404.

3 Jensen TK, Gulbrandsen W, Mossige S, *et al.* Reporting possible sexual abuse: a qualitative study on children's perspectives and the context for disclosure. *Child Abuse Negl.* 2005; **29**: 1395–413.

4 Bolen RM, Lamb JL. Ambivalence of nonoffending guardians after child sexual abuse disclosure. *J Interpers Violence.* 2004; **19**(2): 185–211.

5 Valente SM. Sexual abuse of boys. *J Child Adolesc Psychiatr Nurs.* 2005; **18**(1): 10–16.

6 Tolman DL, Striepe MI, Harmon T. Gender matters: constructing a model of adolescent sexual health. *J Sex Res.* 2003; **40**(1): 4–12.

7 Angelides S. The emergence of the paedophile in the late twentieth century. *Aust Hist Stud.* 2005; **126**: 272–95.

8 Englar-Carlson M. Masculine norms and the therapy process. In: Englar-Carlson M, Stevens MA, editors. *In the Room with Men: a casebook of therapeutic change.* Washington DC: American Psychological Association; 2006. pp. 13–47.

9 Lisak D. Male gender socialisation and the perpetration of sexual abuse. In: Levant RF, Brooks GR, editors. *Men and Sex: new psychological perspectives.* New York: John Wiley & Sons; 1997. pp. 156–77.

10 Craib I. *Experiencing Identity.* London: Sage Publications; 1998. p. 88.

11 Smith AMA, Rissel CE, Richters J, *et al.* Sexual identity, sexual attraction and sexual experience among a representative sample of adults. *Aust N Z J Public Health.* 2003; **27**(2): 138–45.

12 Tacey DJ. *Edge of the Sacred: transformation in Australia.* North Blackburn, Victoria: Harper Collins; 1995. p. 51.

13 Good GE, Sherrod NB. Men's resolution of nonrelational sex across the lifespan. In: Levant RF, Brooks GR, editors. *Men and Sex: new psychological perspectives*. New York: John Wiley & Sons; 1997. pp. 181–204.

14 MacMillan HL, Fleming JE, Streiner DL, *et al.* Childhood abuse and lifetime psychopathology in a community sample. *Am J Psychiatry.* 2001; **158**(11): 1878–83.

15 Jordan JV. Foreword. In: Pollack WS, Levant RF, editors. *New Psychotherapy for Men.* New York: John Wiley & Sons; 1998. pp. xi–xiii.

Chapter 9 Kids and adults that don't tell

1 Hunter SV. Beyond surviving: gender differences in response to early sexual experiences with adults. *J Fam Issues.* 2009; **30**: 391–412.

Chapter 10 Drawing together the threads of resilience

1 McLeod J. *Narrative and Psychotherapy.* London: Sage Publications; 1997.

2 Gergen KJ. *An Invitation to Social Construction.* London: Sage Publications; 1999.

3 Hunter SV. Constructing a sense of self following early sexual experiences with adults: a qualitative research project. *Psychotherapy in Australia.* 2007; **13**(4): 12–21.

4 McCann L, Pearlman LA. Vicarious traumatisation: a framework for understanding the psychological effects of working with victims. *J Trauma Stress.* 1990; 3(1): 131–49.

5 Gill M, Tutty LM, op. cit.

6 Putnam FW, op. cit.

7 Finkelhor D, Berliner L, op. cit.

8 Finkelhor D, op. cit.

9 Herman JL. Complex PTSD: a syndrome in survivors of prolonged and repeated trauma. In: Everly GS, Lating JM, editors. *Psychotraumatology: key papers and core concepts in post-traumatic stress.* New York: Plenum Press; 1995. pp. 87–97.

10 Herman JL. *Trauma and Recovery: the aftermath of violence.* New York: Basic Books; 1992.

11 Chu JA. *Rebuilding Shattered Lives.* New York: John Wiley & Sons; 1998.

12 Masson J. *The Assault on Truth: Freud and child sexual abuse.* Hammersmith: Fontana; 1992.

13 Freud S, Breuer J, op. cit. Vaillant GE. The Wisdom of Ego. Cambridge: Harvard University Press; 1993.

14 Rutter M, Giller H, Hagell A, op. cit.

15 Ross CA. *Dissociative Identity Disorder.* 2nd ed. New York: John Wiley & Sons; 1997.

16 Herckelbach H, Devilly GJ, Rassin E. Alters in dissociative identity disorder: metaphors or genuine entities? *Clin Psychol Rev.* 2002; **22**: 481–97.

17 Robertson RE. The history of dissociative identity disorder. *Undergraduate Psychology Journal.* 2003 (Spring).

18 Ross CA, op. cit.

19 Lynn SJ, Pintar J. The social construction of multiple personality disorder. In: Read RD, Lindsay DS, editors. *Recollections of Trauma: scientific evidence and clinical practice.* New York: Plenum Press; 1997. pp. 483–91.

20 Ibid. p. 487.

21 Herman JL, op. cit. p. 105.

22 Phillips A, Daniluk JC, op. cit.

23 Ullman SE, Filipas HH, op. cit.

24 Phillips A, Daniluk JC, op. cit.

25 Gergen M. Once upon a time: a narratologist's tale. In: Daiute C, Lightfoot C, editors. *Narrative Analysis: studying the development of individuals in society.* Thousand Oaks, California: Sage Publications; 2004. pp. 267–85.

26 Thomas PM. Protection, dissociation, and internal roles: modelling and treating the effects of child abuse. *Rev Gen Psychol.* 2003; **7**(4): 364–80.

27 Lisak D, op. cit.

28 Etherington K. *Narrative Approaches to Working with Adult Male Survivors of Child Sexual Abuse: the clients', the counsellor's and the researcher's story.* London: Jessica Kingsley; 2000.

Chapter 11 Gender differences in the development of narratives of resilience and disclosure

1 Werner EE, op. cit. Riley JR, Masten AS. Resilience in context. In: Peters RDV, Leadbeater B, McMahon RJ, editors. *Resilience in Children, Families, and Communities.* New York: Kluwer Academic/Plenum; 2005. pp. 13–25.

2 Roisman GI. Conceptual clarifications in the study of resilience. *Am Psychol.* 2005; April: 264–5.

3 Riley JR, Masten AS, op. cit.

4 Sidebotham P, Heron J, op. cit.

5 May-Chahal C, Cawson P, op. cit.

6 Sidebotham P, Heron J, op. cit. McCloskey L, Bailey JA. The intergenerational transmission of risk for child sexual abuse. *J Interpers Violence.* 2000; **15**(10): 1019–35.

7 Bolen RM. Attachment and family violence: complexities in knowing. *Child Abuse Negl.* 2005; **29**: 845–52.

8 May-Chahal C, Cawson P, op. cit.

9 Bolen RM, op. cit.

10 Ward E. *Father–Daughter Rape.* London: The Women's Press; 1984.

11 Foster A, op. cit.

12 Apfelbaum ER. And now what, after such tribulations? *Am Psychol.* 2000; **55**(9): 1008–13.

13 Rosenblatt PC. Grief that does not end. In: Klass D, Silverman PR, Nickman SL, editors. *Continuing Bonds: new understandings of grief.* Washington DC: Taylor & Francis; 1996. pp. 45–58.

14 Crossley ML, op. cit.

15 London K, Bruck M, Ceci SJ, *et al.*, op. cit.

16 Alaggia R. Many ways of telling: expanding conceptualisations of child sexual abuse disclosures. *Child Abuse Negl.* 2004; **28**: 1213–27.

17 Jensen TK, Gulbrandsen W, Mossige S, *et al.*, op. cit.

18 Kogan SM, op. cit.

19 Freeman KA, Morris TL. A review of conceptual models explaining the effects of child sexual abuse. *Aggress Violent Behav.* 2001; **6**: 357–73.

20 Rencken RH, op. cit. p. 96.

21 Valente SM, op. cit. Frazier PA, Conlon A, Glaser T. Positive and negative life changes following sexual assault. *J Consult Clin Psychol.* 2001; **69**(2): 1048–55.

22 Gilligan C, op. cit.

23 Welldon EV, op. cit.

24 Tolman DL. *Dilemmas of Desire: teenage girls talk about sexuality*. Cambridge: Harvard University Press; 2002.

25 Taylor JM, Gilligan C, Sullivan AM. *Between Voice and Silence: women and girls, race and relationship*. Cambridge: Harvard University Press; 1995.

26 Lev-Wiesel R, op. cit.

27 Werner EE, op. cit.

28 Craib I, op. cit.

29 Ibid. p. 95.

30 Tacey DJ. p. 51.

31 Kia-Keating M, Grossman FK, Sorsoli L, *et al.*, op. cit.

32 Gill M, Tutty LM, op. cit.

33 Good GE, Sherrod NB.

34 Lusterman D-D. Repetitive infidelity, womanising, and Don Juanism. In: Levant RF, Brooks GR, editors. *Men and Sex: new psychological perspectives*. New York: John Wiley & Sons; 1997. p. 96.

35 Chu JY, Porche MV, Tolman DL. The adolescent masculinity ideology in relationships scale: development and validation of a new measure for boys. *Men and Masculinities*. 2005; **8**(1): 93–115.

36 Tacey DJ, op. cit.

37 Rencken RH, op. cit.

38 Gill M, Tutty LM. Sexual identity issues for male survivors of childhood sexual abuse: a qualitative study. *J Child Sex Abus*. 1997; **6**(3): 31–47.

39 Rencken RH, op. cit. p. 95.

40 Lisak D, op. cit.

41 Ibid.

42 Herman JL, op. cit.

43 Robb C. *This Changes Everything: the relational revolution in psychology*. New York: Farrar, Straus and Giroux; 2006.

44 Gilligan C, op. cit.

45 Lisak D, op. cit.

Chapter 12 How to heal relational injuries caused by childhood sexual experiences

1 Lieb RJ, Kanofsky S. Toward a constructivist control mastery theory: an integration with narrative therapy. *Psychother Theor Res Pract Train*. 2003; **40**(3): 187–202.

2 Erickson EH. *Childhood and Society*. 2nd ed. New York: WW Norton & Company; 1963.

3 Bowlby J. The making and breaking of affectional bonds. *Br J Psychiatry*. 1977; **130**: 201–10.

4 Finkelhor D, op. cit.

5 Herman JL, op. cit.

6 Robb C, op. cit.

7 Fleming J, Mullen P. Long term effects of child sexual abuse. *Issues in Child Abuse Prevention*, Australian Institute for Family Studies. 1998; **9**(11).

8 Gold SN, Lucenko BA, Elhai JD, *et al*. A comparison of psychological/psychiatric symptomology of women and men sexually abused as children. *Child Abuse Negl*. 1999; **23**(7): 683–92.

9 Staller KM, Nelson-Gardell D. 'A burden in your heart': lessons of disclosure from female preadolescent and adolescent survivors of sexual abuse. *Child Abuse Negl.* 2005; **29**: 1415–32.

10 Ibid.

11 Skinner J. *Coping with Survivors and Surviving.* London: Jessica Kingsley; 2000.

12 White M. Narrative therapy and externalising the problem. In: Gergen M, Gergen KJ, editors. *Social Construction: a reader.* London: Sage Publications; 2003. pp. 163–8.

13 McLeod J, op. cit.

14 Fine M, Weis L, Weseen S, *et al.* For whom? Qualitative research, representations, and social responsibilities. In: Denzin NK, Lincoln YS, editors. *The Landscape of Qualitative Research: theories and issues.* Thousand Oaks, California: Sage Publications; 2003. pp. 167–207.

15 Worrell M. Working at being survivors: identity, gender and participation in self-help groups. In: Reavey P, Warner S, editors. *New Feminist Stories of Child Sexual Abuse: sexual scripts and dangerous dialogues.* London: Routledge; 2003. pp. 210–15.

16 Warner S, op. cit. Phillips A, Daniluk JC, op. cit.

17 Phillips A, Daniluk JC, op. cit.

18 Australian Institute of Health and Welfare. *Child Protection Australia 2003/04.* Canberra: Australian Institute of Health and Welfare; 2005.

19 Tilbury C. Child protection services in Queensland post-Forde Inquiry. *Children Australia.* 2005; **30**(3): 10–16.

20 Corby B. *Child Abuse: towards a knowledge base.* 3rd ed. Maidenhead: Open University Press; 2006.

21 Bowlby J. *A Secure Base: clinical applications of attachment theory.* London: Tavistock/ Routledge; 1988.

22 Thomas PM, op. cit.

23 Shamai M, Levin-Megged O. The myth of creating an integrative story: the therapeutic experiences of Holocaust survivors. *Qual Health Res.* 2006; **16**(5): 692–712.

24 Gold SN. *Not Trauma Alone: therapy for child abuse survivors in family and social context.* Philadelphia: Brunner/Routledge; 2000.

25 Etherington K. *Trauma, the Body and Transformation: a narrative inquiry.* London: Jessica Kingsley; 2003.

26 Herman JL, op. cit. p. 187.

27 Cousins C. The 'rule of optimism': dilemmas of embracing a strength based approach in child protection. *Children Australia.* 2005; **30**(2): 28–32.

28 Oellerich TD. Rind, Tromovitch, and Bauserman: politically incorrect – scientifically correct. *Sex Cult.* 2000; **4**(2): 67–81.

29 Read J, Agar K, Barker-Collo S, *et al.* Assessing suicidality in adults: integrating childhood trauma as a major risk factor. *Prof Psychol Res Pr.* 2001; **32**(4): 367–72.

30 Paul LA, Gray JD, Elhai JD, *et al.* Promotion of evidence-based practices for child traumatic stress in rural populations: identification of barriers and promising solutions. *Trauma Violence Abuse.* 2006; **7**(4): 260–73.

31 Kottler JA, Carlson J. *The Client Who Changed Me: stories of therapist personal transformation.* New York: Brunner/Routledge; 2006.

Appendix 2 Research methodology

1 Barbour RS. Checklists for improving rigour in qualitative research: a case of the tail wagging the dog? *BMJ.* 2001; **322**: 1115–17.
2 Denov MS. A culture of denial: exploring professional perspectives on female sex offending. *Can J Criminol.* 2001; **43**(3): 303–29.

Appendix 3 Limitations of the research methodology

1 Dorais M, op. cit. p. 179.
2 McLeod J, op. cit.

Index

T - #0655 - 101024 - C0 - 246/174/12 - PB - 9781846193378 - Gloss Lamination